My
Dog
has
Epilepsy
– but lives life to the full!

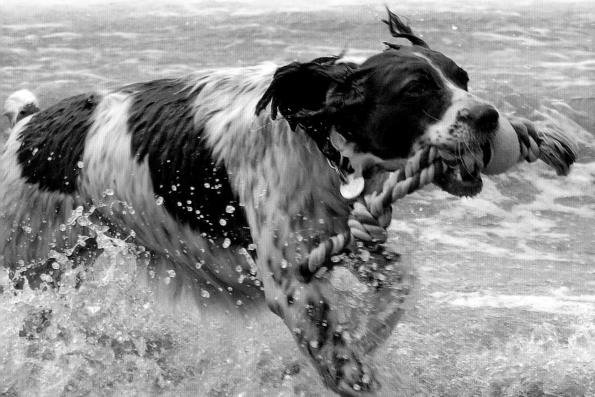

A practical guide for owners

Hubble & Hattie

The Hubble & Hattie imprint was launched in 2009 and is named in memory of two very special Westies owned by Veloce's proprietors.

Since the first book, many more have been added to the list, all with the same underlying objective: to be of real benefit to the species they cover, at the same time promoting compassion, understanding and respect between all animals (including human ones!)

Hubble & Hattie is the home of a range of books that cover all-things animal, produced to the same high quality of content and presentation as our motoring books, and offering the same great value for money.

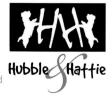

More titles from Hubble and Hattie

Among the Wolves: Memoirs of a wolf handler (Shelbourne)
Animal Grief: How animals mourn (Alderton)
Camper vans, ex-pats & Spanish Hounds: from road trip to rescue – the strays of Spain (Coates & Morris)
Cat Speak: recognising & understanding behaviour (Rauth-Widmann)
Clever dog! Life lessons from the world's most successful animal (O'Meara)
Complete Dog Massage Manual, The – Gentle Dog Care (Robertson)
Dieting with my dog: one busy life, two full figures ... and unconditional love (Frezon)
Dinner with Rover: delicious, nutritious meals for you and your dog to share (Paton-Ayre)
Dog Cookies: healthy, allergen-free treat recipes for your dog (Schöps)
Dog-friendly Gardening: creating a safe haven for you and your dog (Bush)
Dog Games – stimulating play to entertain your dog and you (Blenski)
Dog Sense and CBT - Through your dog's eyes (Garratt)
Dog Speak: recognising & understanding behaviour (Blenski)
Dogs on Wheels: travelling with your canine companion (Mort)
Emergency First Aid for dogs: at home and away (Bucksch)
Exercising your puppy: a gentle & natural approach – Gentle Dog Care (Robertson & Pope)
Fun and Games for Cats (Seidl)
Gymnastricks – targeted muscle training for dogs (Mayer)
Helping minds meet: skills for a better life with your dog (Zulch & Mills)
Know Your Dog – The guide to a beautiful relationship (Birmelin)

Life Skills for Puppies: laying the foundation for a loving, lasting relationship (Zulch & Mills)
Life with a feral dog (Tenzin-Dolma)
Miaow! Cats really are nicer than people! (Moore)
My cat has arthritis – but lives life to the full! (Carrick)
My dog has arthritis – but lives life to the full! (Carrick)
My dog is blind – but lives life to the full! (Horsky)
My dog is deaf – but lives life to the full! (Willms)
My dog has epilepsy – but lives life to the full! (Carrick)
My dog has hip dysplasia – but lives life to the full! (Haüsler & Friedrich)
My dog has cruciate ligament injury – but lives life to the full! (Haüsler & Friedrich)
My Dog, my Friend: heart-warming tales of canine companionship from celebrities and other extraordinary people (Gordon)
No walks? No worries! Maintaniing wellbeing in dogs on restricted exercise (Ryan & Zulch)
Older Dog, Living with an – Gentle Dog Care (Alderton & Hall)
Partners – Everyday working dogs being heroes every day (Walton)
Smellorama – nose games for dogs (Theby)
Swim to recovery: canine hydrotherapy healing – Gentle Dog Care (Wong)
The Truth about Wolves and Dogs: dispelling the myths of dog training (Shelbourne)
Waggy Tails & Wheelchairs (Epp)
Walking the dog: motorway walks for drivers & dogs (Rees)
Winston ... the dog who changed my life (Klute)
You and Your Border Terrier – The Essential Guide (Alderton)
You and Your Cockapoo – The Essential Guide (Alderton)
Your dog and you – understanding the canine psyche (Garratt)

PHOTO CREDITS

The photos have been graciously supplied by individual owners, the author, or, where indicated, external sources.

For post publication news, updates and amendments relating to this book please visit www.hubbleandhattie.com/extras/HH4619

www.hubbleandhattie.com

First published in November 2014 by Veloce Publishing Limited, Veloce House, Parkway Farm Business Park, Middle Farm Way, Poundbury, Dorchester, Dorset, DT1 3AR, England. Fax 01305 250479/email info@hubbleandhattie.com/web www.hubbleandhattie.com ISBN: 978-1-845846-19-0 UPC: 6-36847-04619-4 © Gill Carrick & Veloce Publishing Ltd 2014. All rights reserved. With the exception of quoting brief passages for the purpose of review, no part of this publication may be recorded, reproduced or transmitted by any means, including photocopying, without the written permission of Veloce Publishing Ltd. Throughout this book logos, model names and designations, etc, have been used for the purposes of identification, illustration and decoration. Such names are the property of the trademark holder as this is not an official publication. Readers with ideas for books about animals, or animal-related topics, are invited to write to the editorial director of Veloce Publishing at the above address. British Library Cataloguing in Publication Data – A catalogue record for this book is available from the British Library. Typesetting, design and page make-up all by Veloce Publishing Ltd on Apple Mac. Printed in India by Replika Press

Contents

Acknowledgements, Introduction and Dedication

Acknowledgements

Special thanks are due to Dr Georgina Child, specialist in veterinary neurology at SASH vets in Sydney, Australia, for her expert input, patience and guidance on canine epilepsy. I'd also like to express my gratitude to Cathryn Mellersh and Tom Lewis of the Animal Health Trust charity in Newmarket, Suffolk.

Thanks also go to Dr Holger Volk of the Royal Veterinary College in Hertfordshire; Nick Thompson, the holistic vet in Bath; Richard Allport of the Natural Medicine Centre in Hertfordshire; Jenny Corrall and Sebastien Behr of Willows Referral Services; Julia Robertson of the Galen Therapy Centre; Sally and Ron Askew of EGCBT; Louise Collins of Chief Glen; Eddie and Nicola of Mr Schnorby's, and all at Yappers & Barkers, in Cromer, Norfolk; Dietrich Graf von Schweinitz of the ABVA; Lisa Nickless of the PDSA press office; Rob Fellows of Reiki4dogs; Ken at Norfolk Pet Crematorium; Kylie Baracz of *Dog's Life* magazine; Alex Hurrell of *Eastern Daily Press* (EDP) newspapers, and Hannah of *Dogs Today* magazine.

Finally, I owe a huge debt of gratitude to the marvellous owners who've shared their dog's inspiring stories with me, and have kindly sent me photos of their firmest friends enjoying their life to the hilt. Particularly Pam Cole, who suggested the subject of this book, and whose lovely dog, Bracken – featured on the front cover – is proof positive that an epilepsy diagnosis doesn't have to be the end of your dog's world.

Introduction

Just like humans, dogs can suffer from seizures at some point in their lives, for a variety of reasons. Fortunately, for many, these seizures are one-offs or few-and-far-between, but if they happen frequently then epilepsy – sometimes described as recurrent seizure disorder – is at the root of the problem.

Epilepsy is one of the most common neurological conditions in our furry friends with as many as one in every 20 dogs affected to varying degrees. The condition usually develops before a dog's fifth birthday, and can be more prevalent in certain breeds, although dogs of any age, breed or crossbreed can be epileptic. In the

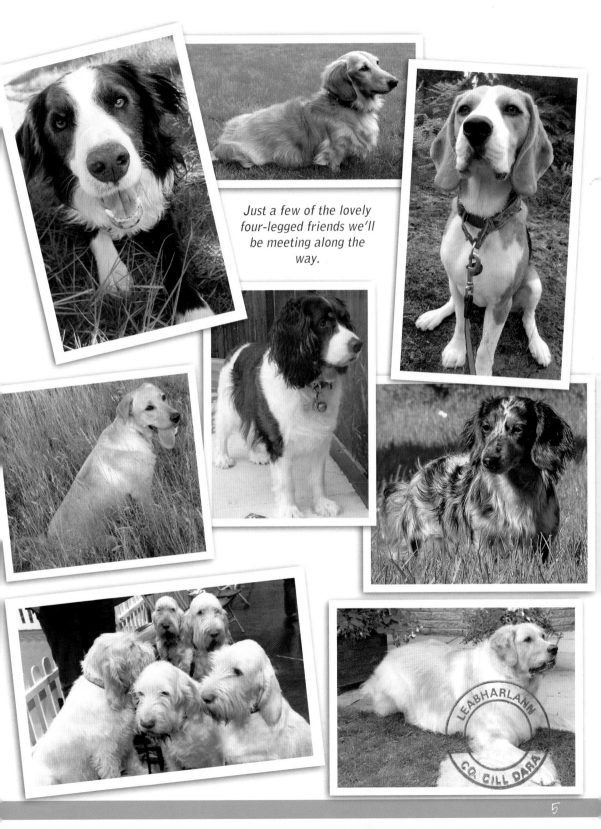

Just a few of the lovely four-legged friends we'll be meeting along the way.

majority of cases, the cause is unknown.

However, with the right treatment, and lifestyle changes where necessary, most epileptic dogs can live a relatively normal life, enjoying all the things they love to do, as before, and our job is to make sure they get the treatment they deserve and all the help they need to cope with the condition.

Whether your dog has just been diagnosed with epilepsy, or has lived with the condition for some time, hopefully, this book will address some of your concerns. With input from leading neurological vets and other experts, topics such as the different types of seizures; why they happen; treatment options; tips for coping; the right diet; complementary therapies, and quality of life considerations, are covered in this practical guide.

It's always worth sharing your stories with other owners by joining a local epilepsy group, or by taking part in one of the increasing number of online forums for specific breeds affected by the disease, which deal with everything from concerns about the effects of conventional drug treatments, to offering helpful advice.

Finally, stay positive: chances are your dog will, and carry on with her life as before, as our heart-warming case histories show.

Dedication
To all the wonderful dogs that have not let epilepsy stand in the way of living their lives to the full. I wish them well.

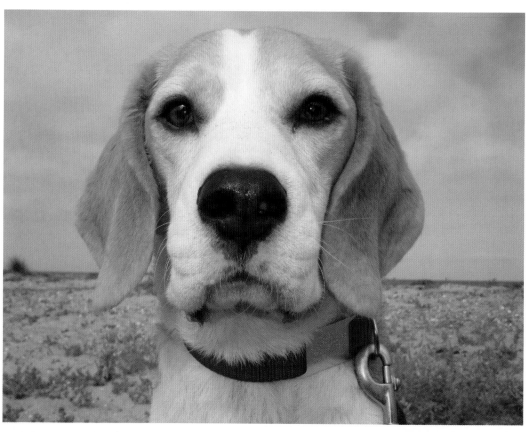

Foreword

Epilepsy, which is simply defined as the occurrence of two or more seizures, is not a disease entity in itself; rather it is a clinical sign usually indicating a forebrain, metabolic or toxic disorder, and is the most prevalent canine neurological disorder. Seizures can be reactive, occurring as a result of a metabolic disorder or poisoning, or symptomatic, resulting, for example, from structural brain disease.

In contrast, the term idiopathic epilepsy refers to recurrent seizures for which no underlying cause can be identified. Dogs with idiopathic epilepsy have an increased risk of premature death compared with the general dog population, and often require lifelong medication to control their seizures and maintain an adequate quality of life. The diagnosis of idiopathic epilepsy is challenging, being one of exclusion, and is made on the basis of normal interictal (between seizure) neurological examination, and exclusion of intracranial (within the brain) and extracranial (outside the brain) causes of seizures by blood and urine tests, magnetic resonance imaging (MRI) of the brain, and cerebrospinal fluid analysis.

Epilepsy can affect dogs of any breed, age and sex. However, it is known to be more prevalent in some breeds than others, and almost certainly has a genetic component in breeds where it is more common than it is in crossbred dogs. In the American Kennel Club's Canine Health Foundation 2013 health poll, epilepsy was ranked 2nd out of almost 300 diseases that worried breeders, with over 40 per cent of breed clubs listing it as a concern.

Although a few rare forms of epilepsy exist that result from mutations in single genes, in the vast majority of breeds epilepsy is thought to have a complex mode of inheritance; meaning it results from mutations in more than one gene. Studies to identify mutations that are responsible for canine epilepsy have enjoyed only limited success to date, and might have been confounded by the inclusion of dogs suffering from seizures for a variety of reasons, rather than just those with a rigorous diagnosis of idiopathic epilepsy.

The Animal Health Trust is investigating the genetic basis of idiopathic epilepsy in several breeds, and routinely asks owners of dogs suffering from seizures to complete extensive questionnaires, including questions about their dog's signalment (how the dog looks and behaves prior to a seizure), diagnostic test results, seizure type/frequency, age of onset and treatment: only dogs with a robust diagnosis of idiopathic epilepsy will be included in the genetic investigations. It is hoped that this rigorous approach to the genetic study of epilepsy will yield positive results soon: the ultimate aim being the development of DNA tests with which breeders can reduce the prevalence of epilepsy in those breeds where it is a problem.

The road to the development of DNA tests for epilepsy will, nevertheless, be a long one, and the insights provided by this book regarding the day-to-day, practical management of epilepsy, how to cope during a seizure, and considerations regarding quality of life will undoubtably represent a wealth of useful information and support for owners of affected dogs.

Cathryn Mellersh, PhD
Head of Canine Genetics
Animal Health Trust, UK

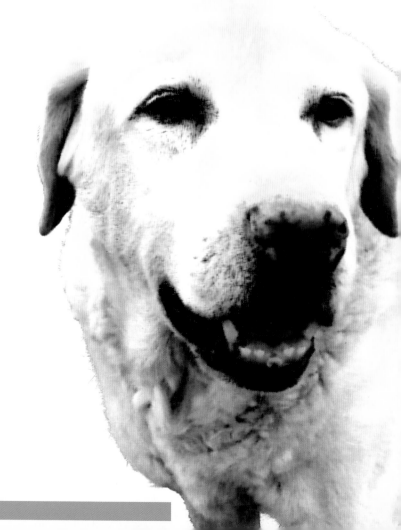

Chapter 1

Canine epilepsy explained

Just like humans, dogs and cats can experience fits, convulsions or seizures at some point in their lives; sometimes just out of the blue. Only when the seizures occur regularly, over a reasonably long period of time – and after other illnesses have been ruled out – will your dog be considered epileptic.

A common condition

Epilepsy is one of the most common neurological conditions among our canine friends: some studies estimate that up to 5 per cent of all dogs – around one in 20 hounds – are affected, and in some breeds this figure could be as high as 15 per cent.

Epilepsy is an unpredictable illness, which can be debilitating and dangerous for your dog if not properly managed. But as separate chapters will show, with veterinary care and the right treatment – alongside a good diet; exercise, and complementary therapies – your dog can still lead a happy, fulfilling life as part of the family.

An historic condition

The ancient Greek philosopher Hippocrates, the father of medicine, believed epilepsy originated in the brain as the result of an imbalance of the four humours (bodily fluids): blood, phlegm, yellow bile and black bile. In our modern world, the condition is often described as an 'electrical storm in the brain.' The disease affects dogs and people in rather the same way.

The canine brain

A dog's brain is a complex mass of nerve tissue, divided into three main areas: the cerebral cortex and its connections (cerebrum); the cerebellum, and the brain stem. The cerebral cortex is the nerve centre, governing learning; memory; hearing; touch; taste, and pain. The cerebrum, which is separated into left and right hemispheres, or lobes, is the part of the brain that malfunctions in epilepsy.

Within the cerebrum are millions of neurons, or nerve cells, which transmit impulses to each other via chemical substances, or hormones, known as neurotransmitters. There are two kinds of neurotransmitters: Inhibitory, which calm the brain and help to create balance, and excitatory, which stimulate the brain. While

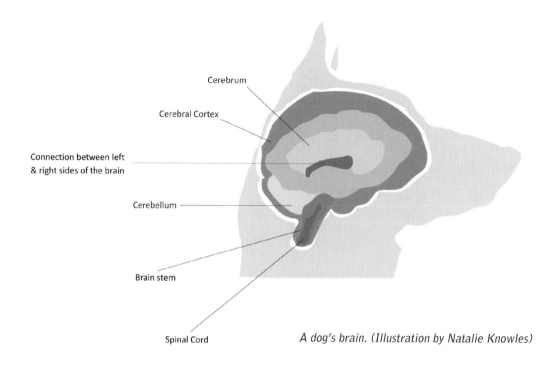

Cerebrum

Cerebral Cortex

Connection between left
& right sides of the brain

Cerebellum

Brain stem

Spinal Cord

A dog's brain. (Illustration by Natalie Knowles)

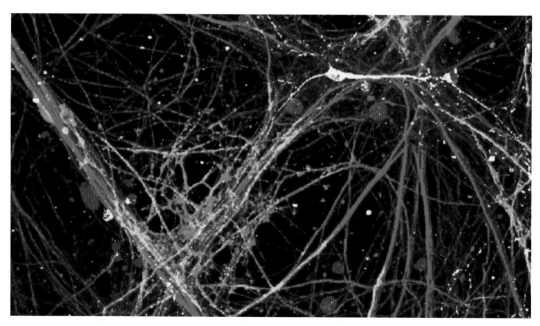

*Neurons. (Courtesy Dr Ragnhildur Thóra Káradóttir, Department of Veterinary Medicine,
University of Cambridge)*

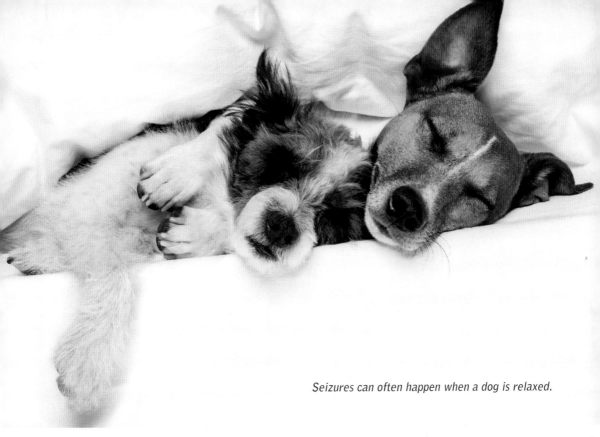

Seizures can often happen when a dog is relaxed.

these hormones usually work in harmony, they sometimes fire off at the same time, effectively overloading the brain; causing a seizure.

When do seizures occur?

Seizures often have no set pattern, and can happen at any time, but often when a dog's relaxed: perhaps having just woken up from a deep sleep. The average seizure lasts for less than two minutes; which probably feels like a lifetime for owners having to watch such an upsetting episode, particularly for the first time. Seizures are broadly divided into two main types: generalised and focal.

GENERALISED

Generalised, or tonic-clonic seizures, are the most severe kind. They happen when the electrical storm appears to arise everywhere in the brain at the same time, making the whole body convulse. A dog will be unconscious, although his eyes will usually stay open.

A tonic-clonic (sometimes referred to as grand mal) seizure might be preceded by a period known as an aura, when a dog's behaviour changes. He might appear anxious, and seek out his owner, or become over-excited.

The start of the seizure is known as the tonic phase, and this lasts for around 30 seconds. Usually a dog's muscles will begin to stiffen; he'll fall to his side with his legs stretched out and his head back. He might make a noise, and his face might begin to twitch. He could drool excessively, and lose control of his bladder and bowel.

During the longer second, or clonic, phase, a dog's limbs will usually begin to jerk; his jaw will be chomping, and his tongue might turn blue.

POST-ICTAL

After the seizure your dog might lie motionless for a while, and then eventually get back on her feet. She might bounce back and seem normal afterwards, although, generally speaking, there's usually a period of post-ictal behaviour after a fit (see chapter 5).

FOCAL SEIZURES

In a focal, or partial, seizure, abnormal electrical activity occurs in only a small area of the brain. These seizures vary in nature, depending on where they've originated in the brain. Dogs could show abnormal movements in only one or more limbs or the face, or behave aggressively during these attacks, or might seem 'not all there,' although still conscious. This type of seizure usually lasts longer than a generalised one, but is thought to cause less damage to a dog's brain.

OTHER SEIZURES

'Absence' or petit mal fits, distinguished in people by staring into space and a reduction in muscle tone, are not commonly recognised in dogs. Dogs of any breed can suffer cluster seizures, when they have one fit, recover, then have another one a few hours' later. If a dog fits continuously with no recovery time in-between, this is known as status epilepticus: an emergency situation requiring immediate veterinary attention.

Why does my dog fit?

There are a number of possible causes, including a brain tumour; a virus; a reaction to chemicals in foods, or perhaps as the result of a vaccination. If a fit occurs when a dog's excited or exercising, this could indicate a heart problem, or low blood sugar. When there's no known cause, the condition is described as idiopathic, or primary, epilepsy. (See chapters 3 & 6.)

Every dog is different

As epilepsy is a complex condition in dogs, there are no hard and fast rules about the course it will take, how your dog will cope with the condition, and how he'll react to any of the drugs he might be taking to help control his epilepsy.

It's a dog's life ...

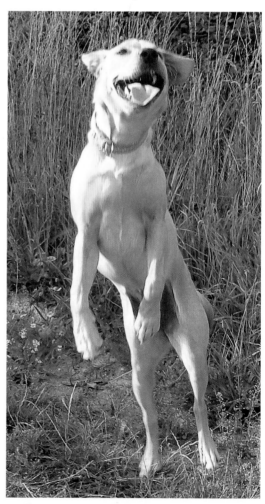

Case history: Inigo

Inigo, 7, is owned by Anne, who says –

"Our boy was two weeks off his fifth birthday when he had his first seizure, and nothing could have prepared us for it. It was, and still is, horrible to see him having a seizure. He's been epileptic for 18 months now, so it is early days yet compared to other dogs.

"His seizures usually last for only a short duration (less than a minute: we have a stopwatch), but always feel like ages to us. When he comes round (if he does not go into another seizure immediately), he is usually blind, so we let him sniff us so he feels safe. We then give him a small amount of ice cream and a couple of drops of Bachs Rescue Remedy to get his blood sugar level up and calm him.

"Each recovery time is different. Sometimes he comes around quickly and is hyper, wanting to play; sometimes he paces/stumbles around and around not settling, walking into things, and sometimes he just goes to sleep. We are battling at present with cluster seizures, and have just tweaked the dose of phenobarbitone to see if we can get him out of this.

"We are lucky in that he usually only seizes every 18-20 days – we can live with that – but the clusters we want to avoid. Hopefully, this will work, but we have learnt quickly that there are no hard and fast rules with canine epilepsy, and it varies from dog to dog. One size definitely does not fit all!

"All in all, I do not think that we will ever get used to the seizures. The only good thing is we believe that he has no recollection of what has happened after a seizure. We treat him exactly the same as he has always been treated: he enjoys daily walks, goes to a dog club every week, and does fun agility in the summer. We just enjoy his company and let him be a dog: after all, he doesn't know he is epileptic!"

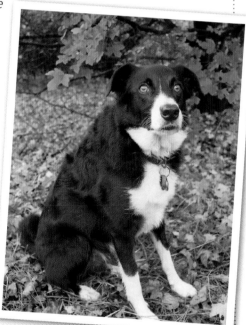

(Courtesy Madelan Gowler)

Should you receive a firm diagnosis of epilepsy, try not to let your natural concerns and fears about what this could mean for your dog overwhelm you, as he will pick up on this, and it will be harder for him to deal with the condition.

Whilst, sadly, there's no cure for epilepsy, and most dogs will have it for life, it's important to adopt a positive attitude, and let your dog live his life as happily and normally as possible. Try to relax, and chances are he'll relax, too, and both of you can get on with your lives, more or less as before.

Case history: Lois

Lois, who's 13, is owned by Jeanne. She says –

"Lois is on phenobarbitone but still fits occasionally. When she gets a seizure she goes into spasm and fails to respond. She doesn't lose control of bodily function like a 'grand mal' type of seizure.

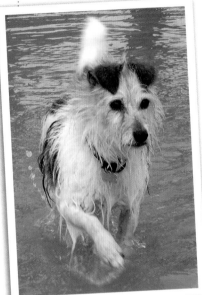

"She appears to feel the onset, but straight afterwards will continue with whatever activity she was engaged in at the time of the fit – be it eating her meal, chasing a ball, or sleeping. Her tastes and weight do not appear to have changed, although we were told when she started medication that she may become more hungry and put on weight. At one time the dose was increased but her fit pattern remained the same and she became very lethargic.

"After this we decided to withdraw medication and for a while her fits were manageable, but then increased to an unacceptable level. We have carefully upped the dosage to a level where she remains a lively Jack Russell, fitting four to 7 times a month."

Case history: Hugo

Hugo, 11, is owned by Joanna, who says –

"Hugo was diagnosed with epilepsy when he was two, and for the last eight-and-a-half years, he has been on 1 x 30mg Epiphen (phenobarbital) twice a day, and 1 x 250mg Epilease (a nutritional supplement with potassium bromide) once a day. I was told to stick to the same time of day for both doses as far as possible, and ideally exactly 12 hours apart. This we have done and I can't even remember when he last had a fit.

"One of the vets at the practice I use wanted to wean Hugo off the drugs altogether, and suggested we halve the dosage of Epiphen. This isn't an exact science at all because the tablet is so small, but Hugo did have a fit when we tried it. The vet then wanted to castrate Hugo as he said anything that reduced stress would help him. As Hugo was already eight years old, I didn't want to go down that route. And I chose not to continue with that vet, too!

"Hugo has to see the vet every six months for further prescriptions of Epiphen (the Epilease I now buy online from Myvetmeds), and has had regular blood tests to ensure his liver isn't suffering. There is no problem there, and he is actually in very good shape. He walks at least half an hour every day; eats well, and his coat is surprisingly good for an older dog that has been on these drugs for so long."

Chapter 2

A diagnosis: what now?

If your dog is seizing regularly this could mean she has epilepsy; but rather than speculate about what's causing the fits, it's a good idea to take your dog to a vet for a proper diagnosis. The earlier the confirmation of epilepsy – if this is indeed the case – the sooner treatment can begin, and your dog can get her life back on track.

Your role

As you're the closest person to your dog your vet will need to get a clear picture from you of life at home since the seizures started. For example, when did your dog have her first fit; how frequent are they, and are there any possible triggers, such as an allergy, or changes to her diet? You'll probably be asked about your dog's behaviour, and whether this has changed recently: perhaps she's more clingy than usual, or simply not her normal self?

Ruling out other problems

A firm diagnosis of epilepsy will also rule out any other health issues that could be causing the seizures, such as a brain tumour, hypothyroidism, or an infection (see chapter 3).

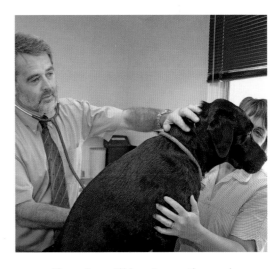

Your dog will be given a thorough examination by a vet ...
(Courtesy British Veterinary Association)

Your dog could be referred to a veterinary neurologist for an epilepsy confirmation, and procedures such as an x-ray, MRI (magnetic resonance imaging), or CT (computerisd tomography) scan, might be carried out. A spinal tap, where a needle is inserted into the lower part

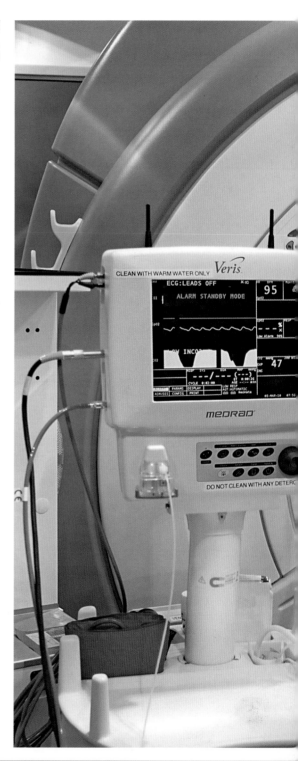

... which may include a scan – such as an MRI – to help diagnose the cause of his seizures. (Courtesy Willows Referral Services)

of the spine and fluid removed, could be performed to give a clearer picture of what's happening inside your dog's body – particularly her brain. If epilepsy is diagnosed, blood tests will usually be taken before treatment is prescribed, to check how your dog's liver and kidneys are functioning.

Tips for coping

It might be upsetting to learn that your dog has epilepsy, but there's no need to panic – help is at hand. The seizures can be reasonably well controlled in the majority of cases, and complementary therapies could help, alongside conventional treatment (see chapters 4 & 9).

KEEPING A DIARY

Keeping a diary, or a chart (which you can download from epilepsy websites), is useful for noting the time, place and build-up to a seizure: whether your dog was resting, sleeping or active at the time; the duration of the fit, and how long it took for your dog to recover. This information will also help your vet to form a clearer picture of your dog's seizure pattern.

It's also worth keeping a record of the medication and dosages your dog's taking, along with the results of any blood tests, and changes in your dog's weight, so you have the information to hand.

CHECKING MEDICATION

If necessary, set an alarm, perhaps on your mobile, to remind yourself when the drugs are due, and consider using a pill dispenser to make it easier to check whether or not you've given your dog his pills. Try and

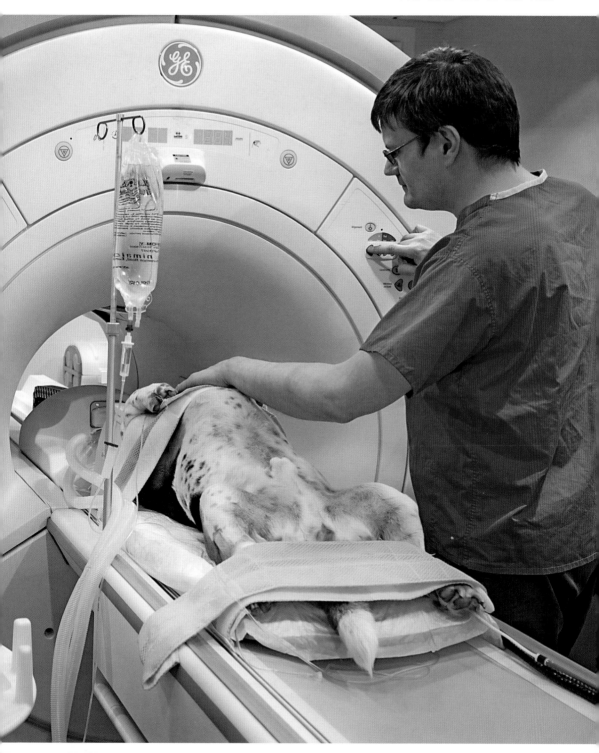

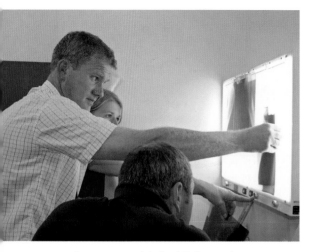

*An x-ray could shed light on the cause
of the seizures.
(Courtesy British Veterinary Association)*

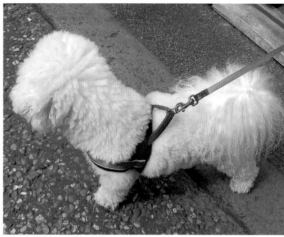

*A harness will help to prevent neck and back
injuries.*

wrap the pills in his favourite treat if he's reluctant to take his medication (as many dogs are).

If you forget to give your dog his pill, give it as soon as possible afterwards, or as your vet advises.

WEARING A HARNESS

A rear or front support harness – for when your dog's on a walk – could reduce pressure on her neck and consequently the risk of injury which could lead to seizures in some cases.

FORUMS

Consider joining an epilepsy group or an online forum, where you can exchange advice – and sympathise – with other owners, and maybe make new friends into the bargain.

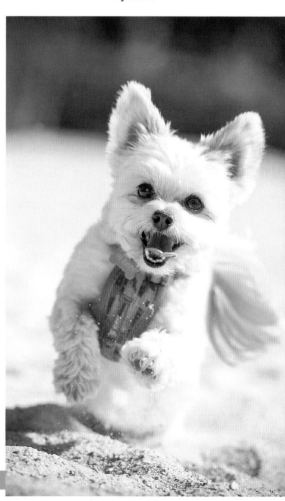

*Peanut has fun in her harness.
(Courtesy EzyDog Australia)*

HOUSEHOLD CLEANERS

Try to rid your home of chemicals such as air sprays/diffusers, cleaning solutions or garden substances to reduce the risk of a reaction. And consider using lavender as a flea or tick repellent, instead of conventional products.

FLOOR SURFACES

If your dog has muscle or joint problems which are aggravated by his anti-seizure medication, he could find certain surfaces, such as slippery tiles or polished wood, challenging, so try putting down some rugs to provide extra grip.

You and your vet

Having a good relationship with your vet is always important, and never more so than if your dog has epilepsy. If there's anything you don't understand about your dog's treatment, say so, and ask for an explanation. And if you're worried about the risks or side-effects of strong drugs, raise the possibility of alternative treatments. Try to find a vet with good experience of epilepsy – and one who cares as much about how you are coping as he does about your dog.

Generally, you'll probably see your vet at least once a year for your dog's annual check – which will probably entail a full physical examination – or more frequently if symptoms worsen.

If you're taking your dog on holiday, or for a trip away from home, it's a good idea to research the nearest emergency vet, just in case you need one.

Epilepsy clinics

Some of the larger veterinary practices, and some veterinary schools, hold regular clinics for dogs whose epilepsy is particularly hard to manage.

The Queen Mother Hospital for Animals,

part of the Royal Veterinary College in Hertfordshire, opened its clinic, the first of its kind in Europe, in 2005. Research continues at the clinic into the functional changes in a dog's brain which lead to epilepsy, and how treatments for the disease can be improved upon.

If your dog's having recurrent seizures and is resistant to standard medication, he could be considered for clinical studies, and perhaps be part of the clinic's ongoing trials for new drugs. Consultations are available weekly; your vet would need to refer your dog.

Typically, during the initial consultation, your dog's history will be discussed with one of the team, and a full clinical and neurological examination will be carried out on your dog's general health, and how his nervous system is functioning. Blood tests, scans and an EEG (electro-encephalography) examination – one of the

Having a check at the Royal Veterinary College. (Courtesy Holger Volk)

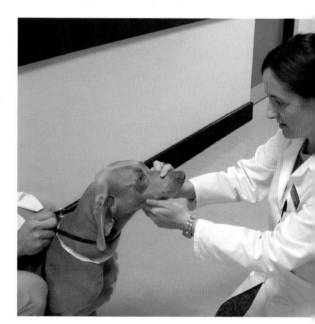

Case history: Otto

Otto, 11, is owned by Veronica, who says –

"I think stress triggers Otto's fits. Not stress as we would think of it, but a case of 'everything not being quite right in his world.' He has always been a very contented dog: well behaved and happy. However, I do remember the first time he had a fit as a puppy, after he had been scratching at a stone in a hard piece of earth. He suddenly shook and went into a sort of trance. I comforted him, but when I picked him up I realised one of his claws was bleeding, and thought it was stress caused by this sudden pain.

"I remember he once had a fit when one of the grandchildren hurt herself and cried; another when we had been out in the car, and came home very late for his meal. He wolfed it down and went outside as usual, but had a fit on the path, which I think was triggered by tummy ache. I also wonder whether fits have been caused by general aches and pains; hunger or thirst.

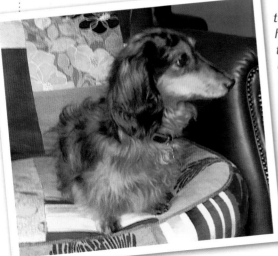

Otto is doing well.

"However, some really good news! After Otto's last annual check, the blood test showed a dramatic improvement. The vet had discussed Otto with a colleague, who said that this sometimes happens as the dog gets older. As a result, Otto now has only half a pill (he was taking 15mg of phenobarbitone every morning), together with half a high strength joint pill.

"He has not had a fit since, and although some mornings he has a snooze, mostly he is bouncing around. He has more energy than he has ever had, and is bright-eyed and happy. We've had two mile walks, and sometimes family walks of four-and-a-half miles, which he has enjoyed.

"However, we take a library book bag with us and carry him in it when he wants a lift, usually after about two miles, then alternately carry him for half a mile, then walk. He seems to sense when the last mile is reached and strides out in front with the children."

few diagnostic tests on the function of the cerebral cortex (see chapter 1) – could be carried out, too.

The role of stress

Some dogs react badly to loud noises, or to people being angry, noisy or aggressive around them, and some owners believe similar stressful situations could trigger a fit, so it's worth trying to make your dog's environment as calm and relaxing as possible. A few drops of lavender and essential oils, diluted with a little water and applied behind your dog's ears, perhaps at bedtime, could help him to relax, for example.

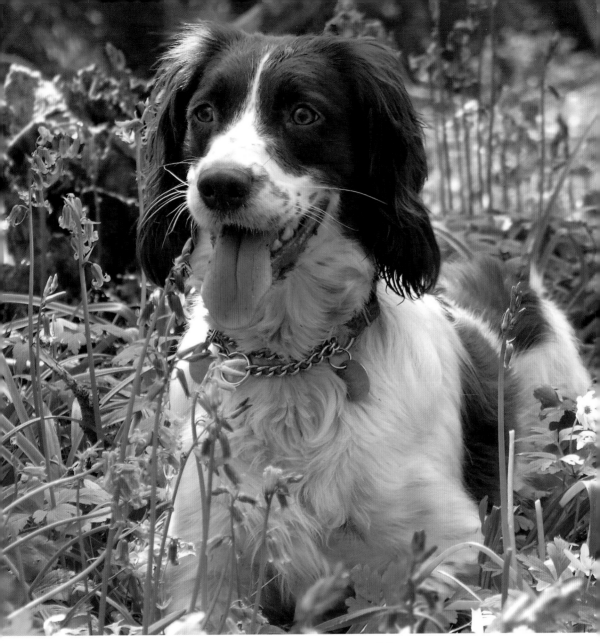

Bracken is living her life to the full.

Phyllis Croft Foundation

The Phyllis Croft Foundation, a charity named after the late Dr Phyllis Croft, who devoted her life to the study of epilepsy and brain disease, supports people caring for dogs with epilepsy.

And remember ...

Try to treat your dog as normally as possible. He won't sit around worrying about his epilepsy, so why should you?

Chapter 3

Causes and triggers

Just why some dogs have seizures isn't always clear, and sometimes there's no obvious explanation. One owner told me her lovely Labrador would suddenly have a seizure whenever he walked past the tv when it was switched on. (She couldn't recall which programme was being broadcast at the time.) And another owner's Springer Spaniel occasionally had a seizure in humid weather. Some owners believe seizures could even be triggered by a full moon.

As a rule, dogs have fits because of certain abnormalities outside of their brain (extracranial) or because of a primary brain defect (intracranial). Seizures can happen because of a brain tumour: a condition known as acquired or symptomatic epilepsy. Sometimes fits have no known cause, which is described as idiopathic – or primary – epilepsy.

Toxins

Seizures can also occur in dogs as a reaction to a range of toxins, including poisons, flea and tick preventives, anti-freeze, insecticides, and paint products. Your dog could also take exception to certain foods, or might have a fit if he's dehydrated. Before making a firm diagnosis or prescribing treatment, your vet will need to know if your dog's been exposed to certain chemicals or foods that could account for the convulsions.

Lyme disease

Seizures can also be caused by Lyme disease: a bacterial infection which affects dogs and humans, and is caused by a bite

Dogs can be allergic to certain foods.

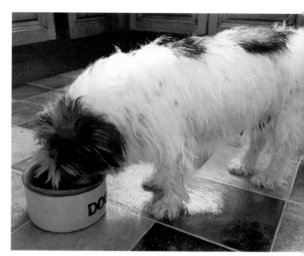

from an infected tick, usually from a deer. It's generally not a serious problem for dogs, and in the majority of cases can be treated effectively with antibiotics.

Distemper

Canine distemper, a contagious and potentially serious viral illness which tends to affect unvaccinated puppies and older dogs, produces fever and dehydration, and can result in seizures as it affects a dog's nervous system in the later stages.

Vaccinations

Whether or not vaccinations can cause health issues is the subject of much debate among owners. As with humans, vaccinations can have side-effects in a very small percentage of cases: it's thought that a vaccination can spark an autoimmune reaction which can lead to secondary swelling in the brain, and seizures in some instances.

Hormone imbalances

When your dog's metabolism is not in tip-top condition, with hormones out of balance, seizures could result. Hypothyroidism, a common hormonal imbalance in dogs, whereby their bodies don't produce enough thyroid hormone, is one example. Although there is no proven link, in one study, three-quarters of the dogs with hypothyroidism had a history of seizures. In female dogs with primary epilepsy, seizures might be first seen, or are worse, when in season (oestrus).

Some dogs with low blood sugar (hypoglycaemia); low blood calcium (hypocalcemia); or high blood potassium (hyperkalemia) can experience fits. Your vet will recommend blood tests to determine whether any of these metabolic conditions are causing the seizures.

Liver disorders

If the liver is not doing its job of eliminating toxins effectively, and there is a build-up in the bloodstream, a dog could develop a condition known as hepatic encephalopathy, which can cause convulsions.

Acquired epilepsy

Various brain abnormalities, such as a tumour, hydrocephalus (fluid on the brain), or encephalitis (brain inflammation), as well as head injuries or traumas, will put pressure on the delicate tissue in your dog's brain. The result is usually seizures and other neurological problems, although these might not develop for years to come in some cases.

These abnormalities are generally the first conditions to be ruled out by your vet, usually through diagnostic testing such as an MRI scan, as a possible cause of the convulsions. If one of these abnormalities turns out to be at the root of your dog's seizures, your dog will be diagnosed

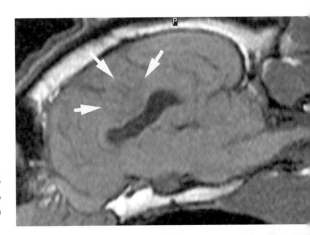

MRI scan showing a tumour. (Reproduced with permission from the BSAVA Manual of Canine and Feline Neurology, 4th edition. © BSAVA)

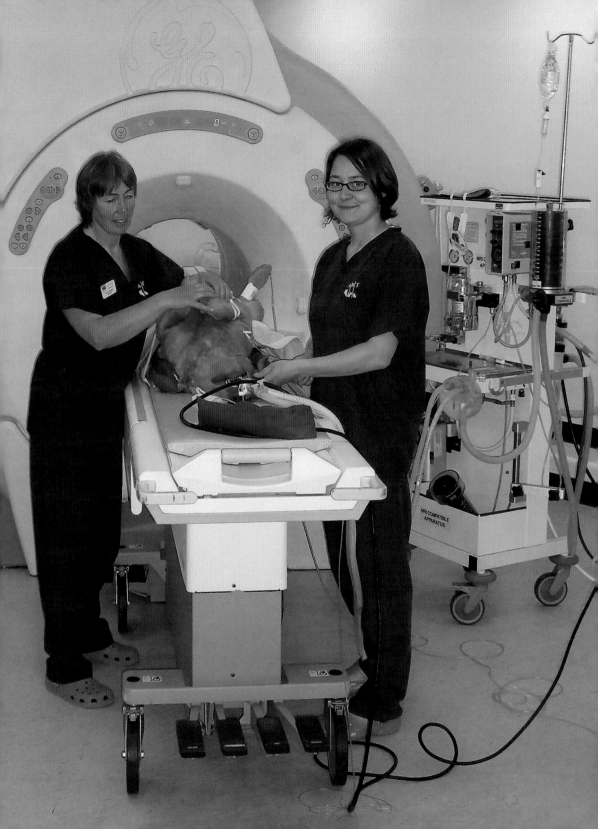

A dog being scanned. (Courtesy Animal Health Trust)

as having acquired – or symptomatic – epilepsy.

While only a small percentage of seizures in younger dogs is caused by tumours, older dogs are more susceptible. Dogs who have their first seizure after their 7th birthday have a 50 per cent chance of suffering a brain tumour.

Idiopathic epilepsy

Idiopathic – or primary – epilepsy is the term applied when there is no known cause for your dog's seizures, aside from a genetic link among some breeds (see chapter 6). It's the most common form of epilepsy. Dogs who have their first seizure when they are under five years old – and particularly between the ages of one and three – are more likely to have this form of epilepsy, although it can affect dogs before they are six months old, or after their third birthday.

This Jack Russell had his tumour removed. (© Sebastien Behr, Willows Referral Services)

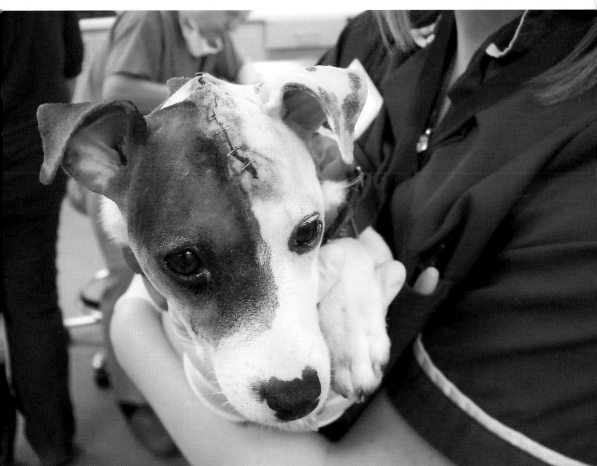

Case history: Dulcie

Dulcie lived until she was 14, and was owned by Dominique. She says –

"Dulcie suddenly started fitting when she was twelve-and-a-half. She would be lying on the sofa next to me, and would suddenly shake from head to toe, with her mouth slightly open. She seemed surprised by it all – and didn't seem to like it one bit. (My other dog, Daisy, didn't seem to be bothered by it at all.) I was frightened and scared, and didn't have a clue what was happening. Dulcie hadn't fitted before and always seemed healthy. She would seize at least once a day, sometimes more, and would always seem to fit in the evening, but, of course, she could have been fitting at other times when I wasn't around.

"We took Dulcie to see our vet, who said it was probably a brain tumour, and that it wouldn't be a good idea for her to have an operation at her late age. I knew he was being practical but the word 'tumour' scared me, and I did wonder about pushing to have it removed, but I knew the vet was right.

"He prescribed a low dose of phenobarbital, which was effective in controlling the fits, and she only had the odd one. I didn't want her to have too much medication, so I was glad the pheno was working. But she seemed dopey all the time: her bright eyes were now dull and she looked vague. She wasn't our bossy Dulcie any more, and about a year-and-a- half later we decided the kindest thing was to put her to sleep."

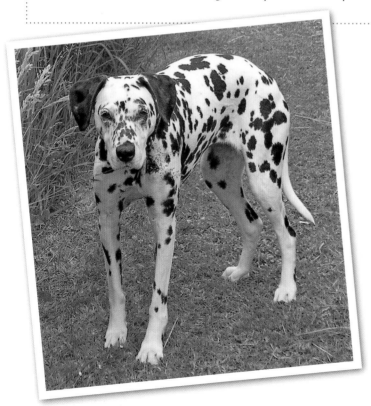

Case history: Bracken

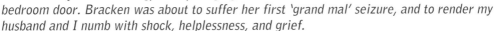

Bracken is 7, and owned by Pam. She says –

"Bracken was, to all intents and purposes, my dream puppy: intelligent, pretty and biddable – everything I could have hoped for! We were going to do so much together, including agility and heel-work to music, but this was all to suddenly change one freezing December night when she was 15 months old, and we were woken at 5.30am by our other dog, Mara, banging on our bedroom door. Bracken was about to suffer her first 'grand mal' seizure, and to render my husband and I numb with shock, helplessness, and grief.

"The next morning our vet performed a raft of blood tests, and was hopeful that this would be a one off as it had coincided with a power surge, and there was also no sign of any clinical illness. After three months of normality, Bracken suffered two more seizures within 48 hours, and she was diagnosed with idiopathic epilepsy at the age of 18 months. I was heartbroken and terrified. Our lovely vet, however, gave me the best piece of advice I have ever received in that we should treat Bracken as a normal dog, as she certainly would not sit around worrying about when she might have another fit: Bracken would just get on with life ... and so should we.

"Then Bracken suffered her first cluster fits early in 2011, and suddenly the fear and helplessness were back with a vengeance. Our vet added potassium bromide to the phenobarbital she'd prescribed to stabilise the clusters, which worked, but had the devastating side-effect of ataxia [loss of balance/co-ordination] in the hind quarters. However, after careful adjustment of the bromide dose and regular hydrotherapy, the ataxia has now all but disappeared, and her mobility is, to all intents and purposes, normal. So it's not the end of the world!

"Bracken still has fits, but we are aware of the triggers and try to avoid them. We'll probably never know what caused her epilepsy, as it could have been several things, from a bad reaction to her first booster, or the anaesthetic when she was spayed, to a knock on the head when a puppy. She has a happy and full life, although I won't pretend it is easy: we try not to dwell on this and simply concentrate on ensuring Bracken enjoys life to the full – for however long that may be."

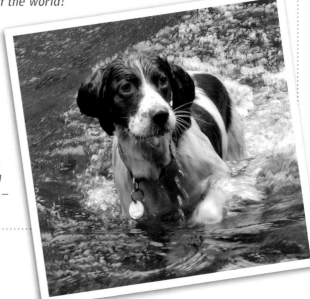

Chapter 4

Treatment options

In an ideal world a cure for epilepsy would be waiting just around the corner, but until this magic bullet is discovered, it's a case of finding the best way to manage this distressing condition in our canine friends.

The current treatment options remain frustratingly limited for owners and vets alike: the choice of drugs is narrow; they don't always work as effectively as they might, and can cause intolerable side-effects in some dogs. Whilst it's unusual for any dog with epilepsy to become seizure-free, even with treatment, on a positive note most dogs respond well to drug therapy, and can experience a reduction of 60-80 per cent in their seizure frequency.

Standard medication

Generally, treatment isn't necessary if your dog has a seizure frequency of less than once a month. When the incidence is higher, anti-convulsant medication is usually prescribed soon after an epilepsy diagnosis, and the two most commonly-used drugs are phenobarbitone (phenobarbital), and potassium bromide, which can be taken in liquid or capsule form.

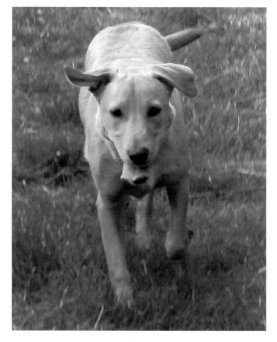

Most dogs with epilepsy experience a reduction in seizure level once they begin their medication.

PHENOBARBITONE (PB)

This is considered to be the most effective drug in reducing seizures (ideally to less than one a month), and in stopping their progress, in around two-thirds of cases of idiopathic epilepsy. Most dogs will be started on a low dose of around 2-3mg per kilo of body weight; although the dose could be higher in severe cases (if not controlled at lower doses). As this drug is processed by the liver, regular blood tests will be necessary to reduce the likelihood of liver damage.

POTASSIUM BROMIDE (KBR)

As potassium bromide has no effect on the liver, it's considered the most appropriate treatment for dogs with existing liver damage. A loading dose might be necessary for dogs with frequent seizures, or when phenobarbitone has to be withdrawn rapidly because of liver disease. It can take up to four months to be fully effective.

KBr might be prescribed by your vet as an 'add-on' if convulsions are not well-controlled with phenobarbitone alone. Twice-daily dosing is generally recommended, as dogs cannot tolerate too much salt in their gastrointestinal tract in one go. On average, a maintenance dose of potassium bromide is 20-30mg per kg of body weight.

PEXION®

This newer drug contains imepitoin, and acts by suppressing electrical activity in the brain, and activating GABA (gamma-aminobutyric acid) receptors. This is a human drug that has moved over to the canine world, and is believed to be better tolerated, with fewer severe side-effects, particularly on a dog's liver, than phenobarbitone.

KEPPRA®

For some dogs, phenobarbitone and potassium bromide might not be enough to control seizures, or their side-effects might not be well tolerated, so your vet might suggest adding Keppra® (levetiracetam) to the mix for greater effect.

VALIUM®

Benzodiazepines such as Valium® might also be prescribed to be administered into your dog's rectum during a seizure.

A lifelong commitment

It often takes a few months to get the dose just right for your dog, and he'll probably need to take this medication for the rest of his life. Although the seizures are unlikely to be eliminated completely with treatment, the fits should be less frequent, hopefully.

The prescribed medication should be taken every day, at roughly the same time, and ideally with food. If the drugs are suddenly stopped, your dog could fit.

Cluster seizures (more than two seizures in 24 hours) are the most challenging to manage, and treatment needs to begin early after diagnosis. The sooner the treatment begins, the better the chance that the seizures can be controlled.

Visits to your vet

As a rule, you're likely to pay a visit to your vet around twice a year after diagnosis, or more often if symptoms worsen. Your dog will need to be assessed regularly to make sure the dosage she's taking is not too high, or too low, and your vet will want to conduct regular blood tests for liver and kidney function to minimize the chances of a reaction to a particular drug, or long term damage.

Kindling

Sometimes the more seizures a dog has, the more likely he is to do so again, as though the brain becomes 'wired' to fits – described as kindling - although this has

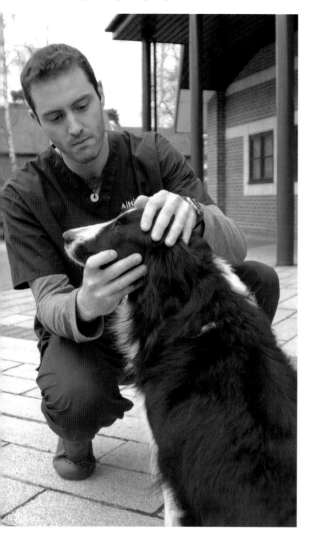

*Your dog's likely to visit a vet around twice a year for check-ups.
(Courtesy Animal Health Trust)*

not been proven. Early intervention with drug treatment could help to prevent this.

Side-effects

No drug is without side-effects, and sometimes these can be serious, particularly if used over the long term and taken in high doses, and this might seem a high price to pay to keep seizures under control. Luckily, many epileptic dogs lead normal, happy lives on their drug treatments, with few side-effects, and any they do experience usually reduce or disappear after the first few weeks, although they could last longer if the medication dose is high. Common side-effects include reduced energy, appearing zombie-like, and ataxia (loss of co-ordination).

Always raise any concerns you have with your vet, and discuss whether there's an alternative drug which might have fewer side-effects, but still keep the symptoms under control. Every dog is different, and some drugs might work better than others for your dog, so it could be a case of trial and error at the start of treatment.

When treatment isn't effective

Although some dogs will continue to experience severe seizures, and require intensive medical management despite daily medication, an increase in the number and severity of seizures doesn't always mean the disease is getting worse. Sadly, some 20-30 per cent of epileptics

continued page 33

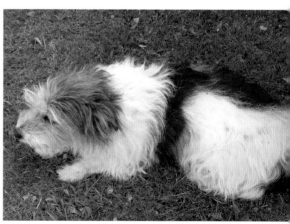

Epilepsy medication can cause lethargy.

Case history: Lula

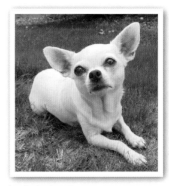

Lula, 7, is owned by Sue who says:

"Lula was diagnosed with idiopathic epilepsy when she was one, and was prescribed phenobarbital and potassium bromide. It's a difficult juggling act between preventing the seizures and dealing with the side-effects of the medication, and it took a while for the meds to work and then to stabilise her. She continued to fit about once every two weeks (sometimes more), and we were grateful if we went a month without a seizure. We tried ocular compression and ice packs to cool her down, and kept a log of the fits. I believe these methods helped as we saw a reduction of her seizing time. We had a two-year period of no seizures, and I thought that she was cured – wishful thinking.

"Lula had regular medication checks, and every six months would have bile acid tests. She was okay for a while, and then had some extremely high results. She developed severe ataxia; her liver was struggling, and the vet suggested we reduce the phenobarbital, but she started to seize so we've decided to keep her on the higher level of meds, and we're tackling her liver problems with a liver supplement called Samylin. The last results were quite good and we're hoping the next ones come back even better.

"We enjoy dog shows, and fun agility in the garden, and I'm no longer fussing over her as if she'll break. I've accepted she needs to be treated as a normal dog, not an intensive care patient."

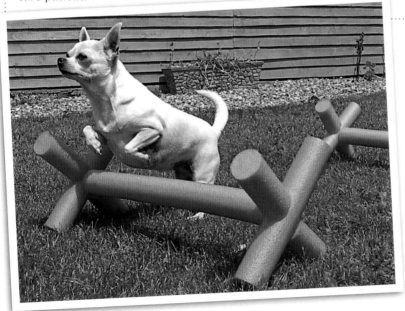

Case history: Shani

Shani is 7, and owned by Jean. She says:

"We've had Shani [rhymes with rainy] since she was eight weeks old. Two weeks after arriving, Shani vomited, but we thought nothing of it as it's quite common in puppies. Then, when she was nine months old she had a 'strange' episode, where she was staggering, and then suddenly went very limp, which frightened my husband and I. She was fine again after about five minutes.

"She continued to vomit every two weeks but, by this time, she had started to run to one of us before it happened – she obviously knew she was going to be sick. It graduated to where she would sometimes suddenly urinate, as if she just had to, and couldn't help it.

"When she was 14 months old she had a grand mal, but it was some time before she had another seizure. Then they became frequent, and Shani was diagnosed with idiopathic epilepsy. Another of our dogs, Sami, had died of phenobarbital-induced liver disease, and we hadn't wanted to give Shani pb, but the fits were too frequent not to. We also had rectal diazepam to administer at the start of a seizure.

"She was seizure-free for three months, but then they started again so gabapentin was added to the phenobarbital. Shani started to seize weekly again a few weeks later, and we increased the pheno. She is only on a low dose, 22.5mg, but weighs just 9lb (4kg). Shani also takes Epitaur, a nutritional supplement.

"After the increase in phenol, Shani went for 66 weeks without a seizure. She then had a reaction to a flea product, and had one seizure a month for the next three months. A few months ago Shani had had a few fits together, and Gail, my vet here in Scotland, wanted to add Libromide (Kbr), so we did. Shani has now been 31 weeks seizure-free and is doing very well.

"I know that Shani is not nearly as bad as so many dogs, and I am grateful for that. Also, in a small dog, the seizures don't seem as bad because they are not magnified as they are in a large dog, so I can put her on my knee, administer the rectal valium, and hold her until it is over."

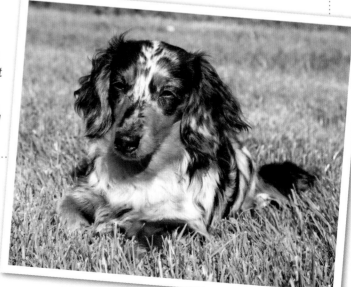

will become resistant to treatment, which might fail for several reasons: perhaps because doses are missed; a dog spits out the tablets or refuses to take the liquid, or has a tummy upset, preventing the drug from being absorbed. The sodium chloride (salt) content of your dog's diet will affect the concentration of potassium bromide.

Controlling costs

Prescription drugs can be expensive, and it's usually cheaper to buy the drugs online, rather than from your veterinary practice. Make sure you use a reputable online site which insists on a valid prescription. (Your vet will be able to supply this, although there's likely be a charge.) It's also worth investing in a good pet insurance plan to cover most (or all) of the costs of treating your dog.

Brain-splitting surgery

Dogs seizing up to ten times a day, even on medication, whose quality of life is poor, have undergone surgery, known as Corpus Callosotomy, to split the connection between the right and left sides of the brain.

Performed by leading veterinary surgeon Dr Charles Kuntz, now based at Southpaws Veterinary Surgery in Victoria, Australia, the surgery has been successful in reducing the number of seizures in some cases, but, as with all operations, isn't without risk.

Visit Hubble and Hattie on the web: www.hubbleandhattie.com & www.hubbleandhattie.blogspot.co.uk
• Details of all books • Special offers • Newsletter • New book news

33

Chapter 5

What to do during a fit

There's a lot to think about when it comes to managing your dog's epilepsy, and knowing what to do when your dog has a fit is one of the most important aspects. First aid knowledge is vital in keeping your dog as injury-free as possible during an attack.

While most seizures last a comparatively short period of time (between 30 and 90 seconds), this may well seem like a lifetime for you, the owner; especially when your dog has his first fit. Over time, however, you'll become well aware of the signs that your dog is about to have a seizure, and how to react. The important thing to remember is to stay as calm as you can, however difficult that might be, and this will become easier over time, too.

Of course, you might not always be around when your dog seizes, so it's a good idea to think ahead, and make sure the area is as safe as possible before you leave home, or take your dog with you if you can.

Risk of injury

One of the obvious signs a dog is about to fit is a change in his usual behaviour: he might be more clingy, or hyper-active, or could look 'not all there.' When you see this change, try to guide your dog to a safe area, and consider turning off the television set, and some of the lights, if possible, to create a calmer, more restful atmosphere.

How to protect your dog, and especially her head, from injury during a fit is, naturally, a concern. Dogs generally have a seizure when resting or sleeping, and if your dog's lying on a hard surface during a fit and her head is jerking, it's a good idea to put something like a towel, a bag or a jumper – whatever appropriate is at hand – under her head to help to protect it.

Safety first

If your dog is lying under a table or near chairs, it's best to move the furniture out of the way, as dogs suffering seizures might become wedged under tables or sideboards, with the accompanying risk of suffocation. Don't put anything in your dog's mouth, or try to hold him down, during a fit.

One owner told me she makes sure that the handles on chests of drawers or cupboards near her dog's basket are padded. It's also a good idea to provide a supportive bed, ideally washable or wipe clean, for your dog to lie on, rather than letting him sleep on your bed, and possibly fall off during a fit.

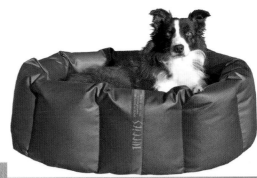

A wipe-clean nest bed. (Courtesy Tuffies)

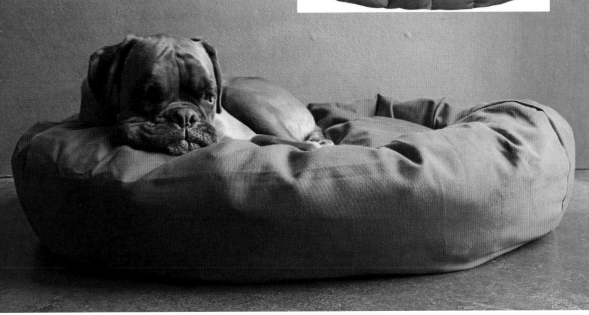

A washable bed is practical. (Courtesy Bone & Rag)

Other measures

Another owner told me her dog rears up when he seizes, so she tries to catch him to prevent him falling back onto something hard. She holds him gently and talks to him all the time, calling his name, and sometimes she sings to him.

Every owner has their own approach: some give their dogs a massage; others Rescue Remedy after a fit, or before they leave their dog at home.

When it's an emergency

Although seizures are generally not life-threatening, if your dog seizes continuously – a condition known as status epilepticus – this is a medical emergency, so immediately take your dog in the car to the vet to prevent risking her life.

After a seizure

The period immediately after a generalised or partial seizure is known as the post-ictal phase, which can vary in length. Some dogs bounce back quickly, and seem perfectly normal after a seizure, almost as if nothing has happened; other dogs might be disorientated for a few days. The length of time it takes an epileptic dog to return to his old self doesn't usually bear any relation to the duration of the fit.

Generally speaking, once the seizure is over, your dog will feel groggy and be unsteady on her feet, so it's important to keep an eye on her to make sure she's okay, without fussing. As fitting uses up a lot of your dog's energy – similar to a human having a work-out at the gym – her muscles could be very sore, and ache quite a lot. She'll also be hungry and thirsty (see chapter 7).

Ice bags

Most dogs become hot during a fit, and applying a bag of ice to the middle of your dog's back (not her neck) could slow the fit or stop it, and possibly also reduce recovery time.

Dog alert

It's well known that dogs can detect illness in humans, so it's no surprise that they can sense conditions, such as epilepsy, in other hounds, too. Sometimes they can act as unofficial alert dogs. One owner told me her dog would bark before the other seized, and it was a challenge to keep him from trying to 'help' the fitting dog. In a similar case, an owner was 'tipped off' by her other dog, giving her time to move the dog who was about to fit to a room with washable floors (in case of incontinence).

Ocular compression (OC)

This is an application of firm but gentle pressure on one or both (closed) eyes during a seizure. It's believed this pressure stimulates the vagus nerve (the 'wandering' nerve that runs from the brain to the abdomen) to release GABA: a neurotransmitter with anti-convulsive effects. It can be effective on occasion.

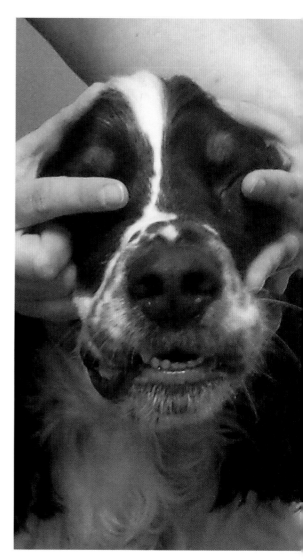

Mr Schnorby receives ocular compression.

Case history: Bella

Tracy, Bella's owner, says –

"Bella was a stray who came to us when she was about four months old. She had cluster seizures, and was started on phenobarbitone, with Keppra® added. She always had the seizures at night while she was sleeping, except once right beside my pool. Luckily, I was nearby, heard her, and ran and scooped her up. Falling in the water would have been fatal while she was fitting.

"You have to take epilepsy seriously, and be organised and ready for seizures. Have a plan and know when you can handle things at home and when to run to the vet. And know where the emergency vet is and how long it would take to drive there. I kept a box on my dresser filled with the brown bottle of diazepam; the needle preloaded on the syringe; a couple of dog training pads to put under her in case of incontinence; a rectal thermometer, and something for under her head.

"Also, I clearly wrote up how may cc/mls to draw up, AND how many mg there were per mls/cc. You need to write down the directions so that, if you are in a panic, you know exactly what to draw up and give. And if that doesn't work, what's the next plan? Ours was two small doses of the rectal diazepam: the second only if the first didn't help. Also, our neurologist gave us oral clonazepam 2mg to be given as two tabs every 8 hours for 24 hours post-seizure to keep her from cluster fitting.

"I also used ice packs to keep her cool, and calmly repeated her name, wiping her face and ears to keep her cool. We usually also had a fan on low, too, just to make sure she didn't overheat (though you don't want to chill them, either). We put a bell on her collar so we always knew where in the house she was, and could keep track of her. She had her favourite spots, and if she varied from the norm, it often meant something was brewing. We did everything we could, but she lost her battle against her illness at 7 – too young to be gone."

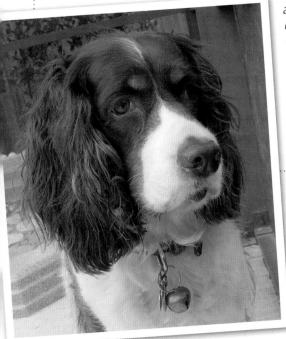

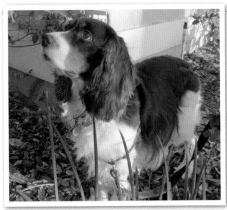

Case history: Tia

Tia, ten, is owned by Carol, founder of CSRBC Cocker Spaniel Rescue in British Columbia, Canada. Says Carol –

"Tia was very ill with a uterine infection when she arrived at the rescue, so she went straight to the vet for surgery. Her siblings had fits, but she was seizure-free at the time, and for the next few months, and we adopted her. Then she had a seizure and the vet put her on phenobarbitone. She's now on 30mg, as well as a supplement thyroid hormone, and milk thistle extract with each meal.

"She was seizure-free for so long, but started seizing in March 2012. I decided to keep a seizure record for her. When she had a seizure in her crate, I lifted her out and put her on a pillow to secure her head. The seizure lasted for about a minute, and she tensed up with minor shaking. She was post-ictal for about 30-45 seconds, then back to normal.

"Her next seizure was six months later, and again lasted for about a minute: she seemed to snap out of it quickly. I applied ocular pressure twice on each eye for a count of ten, and this seemed to slow the seizure. The post-ictal period was about 90 seconds.

"Then, a little later, she went into another seizure. I tried ocular pressure again but it didn't seem to make a difference this time, so I drew up 10mg of diazepam and shot it into her rectum. I didn't document how long that seizure lasted but I remember it not being for long.

"Tia was a wreck three years ago, but she's come a long way, and her pb levels are within the normal range."

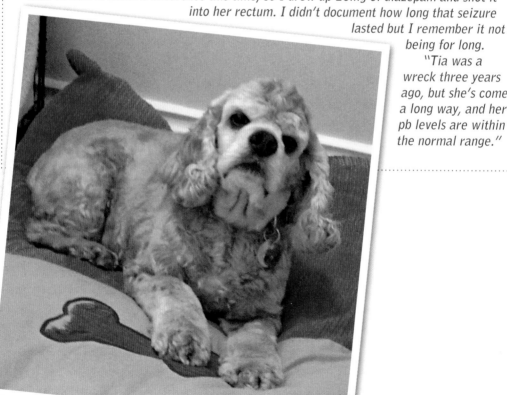

Chapter 6

Breeds affected

While epilepsy can take different forms, the most common is idiopathic or primary epilepsy, which is also referred to as genetic or inherited epilepsy, as it has a genetic basis in certain breeds.

Although any breed, including mixed breeds, can develop idiopathic epilepsy, the condition is believed to be inherited in Beagles, German and Belgian Shepherds, Hungarian Vizslas, English Springer Spaniels, Irish Wolfhounds, Collies, and Dachshunds.

Seizure disorders in other breeds

Irish Setters, Saint Bernards, American Cocker Spaniels, Wirehaired Fox Terriers, Alaskan Malamutes, Siberian Huskies, Welsh Springer Spaniels, Labrador Retrievers, Miniature Schnauzers, Mastiffs and Poodles have a tendency for fitting disorders.

Staffordshire Bull Terriers

Staffies can suffer from a genetic metabolic disorder known as L-2-hydroxyglutaric aciduria, which affects their central nervous system.

Dogs with this condition might have

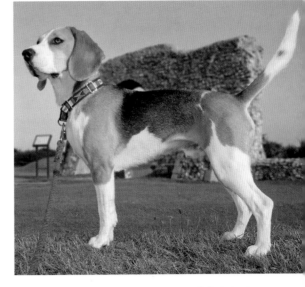

Beagles like Merlin are at risk of developing epilepsy.

epileptic seizures, and their behaviour may be affected as a result.

Popular breeds

Some breeds are always more in demand, and by their sheer weight of numbers

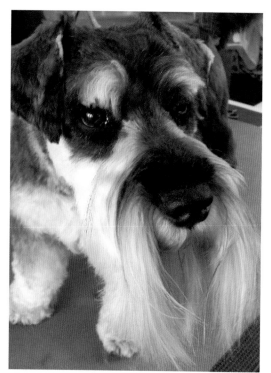

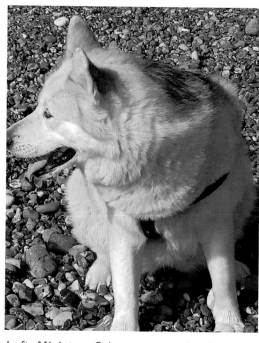

Left: Miniature Schnauzers can develop epilepsy.

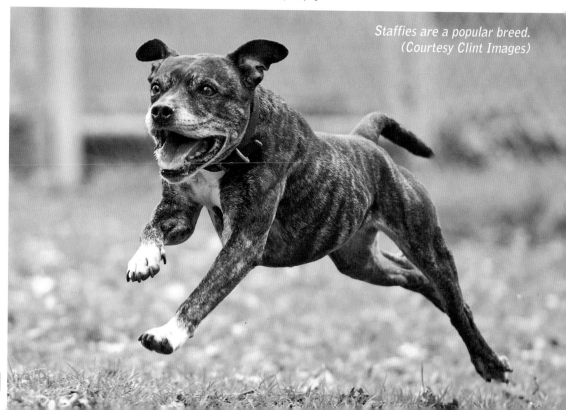

Staffies are a popular breed.
(Courtesy Clint Images)

Left: Kiera the Siberian Husky, luckily, is free of seizure disorders that can affect her breed.

account for more visits to the vet, which could explain why they're considered more prone to diseases such as epilepsy. Dr Georgina Child, a specialist neurological vet at the Small Animal Specialist Hospital (SASH) in Sydney, Australia, says: "In my practice, Boxers, Border Collies, Golden Retrievers, Staffordshire Bull Terriers and Maltese Terriers are over-represented, but are all currently popular breeds as family pets."

Acquired epilepsy

Acquired – or symptomatic – epilepsy,

Max started fitting when he was 18 months old, and was diagnosed with idiopathic epilepsy soon after. His seizures are severe, and he takes phenobarbitone, steroids, and diazepam to try and control them. His owner, Kim, believes epilepsy is badly affecting Max's quality of life.

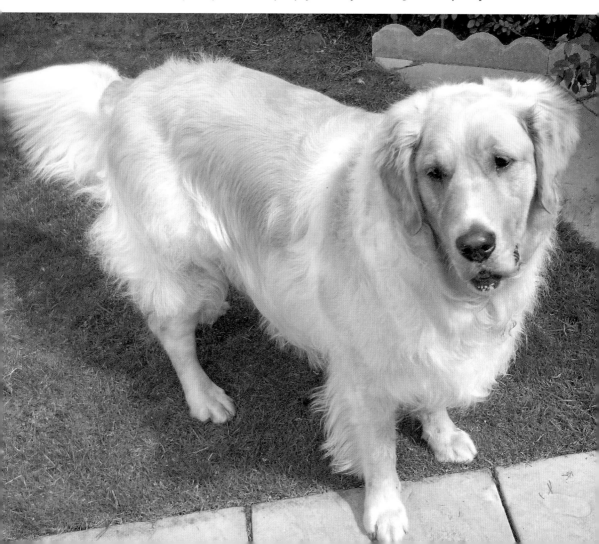

which can develop as the result of a head injury, for example, can be seen in any breed of either sex.

Boys v girls

Male dogs generally have a higher incidence of idiopathic epilepsy than females. Females in season, or pregnant, can experience more seizures. Oestrogen lowers the seizure threshold, and it is not uncommon for bitches to have their first seizure when on heat. A recent study found that whether male or female, dogs that haven't been neutered are more likely to have clusters of seizures – more than two in one day.

Age

Although the age at which a dog develops idiopathic epilepsy – and the type and pattern of seizures he experiences – can differ quite a lot between breeds, dogs with genetic epilepsy are likely to have had their first seizure before their third birthday.

Limited gene pool

There are an estimated 400 breeds of dog worldwide, and around 200 recognised breeds in the UK, with five million pedigree dogs among these different breeds.

While the human population is 'out-bred,' pedigree dogs have a much more limited gene pool to draw on, making the risk of developing inherited diseases, like epilepsy, more likely.

Breeders have a significant role to play in helping to eradicate inherited diseases among our pure-bred faithful friends. Says Dr Child: "While there's nothing you can do to prevent the acquired form of the disease, for genetic epilepsy responsible breeding is the key. All epileptic dogs should be spayed."

The genetics of epilepsy

Genetic factors are estimated to play a role in the development of epilepsy in as many as 40 per cent of dogs with idiopathic epilepsy. It's a complex disease, where some dogs might have one, or several, faulty genes (polygenic) in their DNA, predisposing them to seizures, while others might have an abnormal gene, but won't have seizures. Hopefully, ongoing studies will go a long way toward identifying how inherited epilepsy develops in certain breeds.

Belgian Shepherds

Genetic experts at Helsinki University, working alongside Danish, Swedish, and US researchers on an EU-funded project, have been comparing the chromosomes (thread-like materials which carry the genes in animal cells) of Belgian Shepherds with epilepsy, and healthy 'control' dogs. The research found that a gene in chromosome 37 could increase the risk of developing idiopathic epilepsy seven-fold: a breakthrough that could have an impact on our understanding of how epilepsy develops in other breeds, as well as in humans.

Canine Genetics Centre

The Animal Health Trust (AHT), a leading animal health charity, with support from the Kennel Club Charitable Trust and other funding organisations, has been investigating the genetic basis of canine inherited diseases, such as epilepsy.

The aim of the Centre is to help dog breeders reduce, or eradicate, inherited disease from their breeds, and to design breeding programmes to improve the overall health of the breed, while preserving genetic diversity. Geneticists and veterinary neurologists at the AHT are looking into

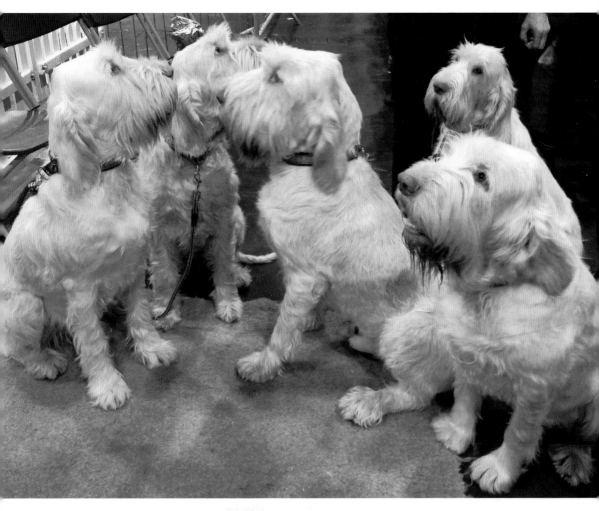

Italian Spinones are taking part in genetic tests at the Animal Health Trust.

idiopathic epilepsy in two breeds: Italian Spinones, and Border Collies.

ITALIAN SPINONES

As part of this ongoing research, breeders and owners are being asked to provide DNA samples, using a simple cheek swab, to help experts at the centre try and identify the mutation(s) that increase a dog's risk of developing idiopathic epilepsy. The aim in the longer term is to develop a DNA test that breeders could use to reduce the prevalence of the disease in this breed.

BORDER COLLIES

The team at the AHT has collected DNA samples from around a hundred affected Border Collies. To increase the chances of success in their research they would like to collect DNA samples from more affected

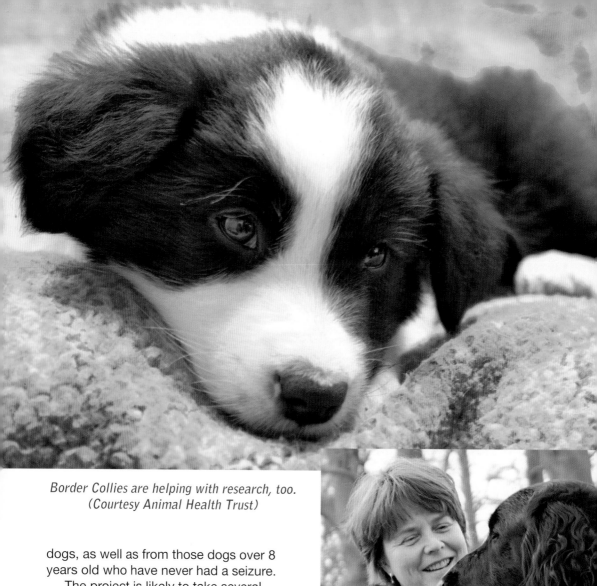

Border Collies are helping with research, too.
(Courtesy Animal Health Trust)

dogs, as well as from those dogs over 8 years old who have never had a seizure.

The project is likely to take several years to complete, and if you own a Border Collie who suffers from epilepsy, and would be happy to donate a DNA sample from your dog (again, using a cheek swab), please contact Bryan McLaughlin (bryan.mclaughlin@aht.org.uk) for a DNA collection kit.

Taking a swab for DNA testing.
(Courtesy Animal Health Trust)

Case history: Goliath

Goliath is 8 and owned by Lynne. She says –

"Goliath is a male Irish Wolfhound who was diagnosed just before his third birthday due to a couple of single seizures, and who began medication just after this birthday, when he had two clusters in two weeks. He was put on phenobarbital, and the dose was adjusted over the next year. We are fairly steady at 105mg twice a day, getting bumped up to 120 or even 150 during the heat of summer, with the blessing of his vet. The dose has resulted in serum levels that are usually below the therapeutic range, but they have kept his seizures down to one every 18-24 months, so this is obviously an effective dose.

"Goliath is a companion pet. He was castrated much too young, and is mildly anxious, and doesn't like change or surprises. But as he has always been like that we don't know whether or not this is related to the epilepsy. His little brother (actually, a great-nephew) is intact, and a perfect example of the breed's temperament.

"Goliath is comfortable with dogs, cats, and most people, but is more self-confident when his little brother is with him, and will do anything if I am with him. The dogs were never trained, but learn quickly and understand what we want of them, and have taught us to understand them, to some extent."

Goliath and little friend.

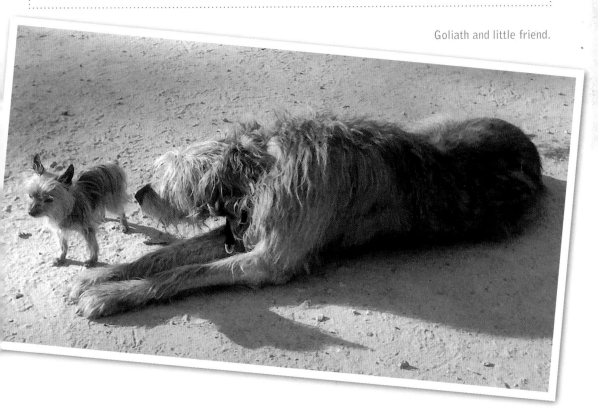

Case history: Tilly

Tilly, 7, is owned by Dr Child, who says –

"Tilly had her first fit when she was two years old. Purebred Border Collies have a known genetic tendency to idiopathic epilepsy, which is often not managed that well with conventional medications, and the breed sometimes becomes resistant to these meds because of a particular gene.

"Tilly was okay on phenobarbitone and potassium bromide for several years, but her cluster seizures continued. She was then put on zonisamide, which is prescribed by vets to treat seizure disorders that don't respond well to standard treatment such as phenobarbitone, or because other seizure medications aren't well tolerated.

"It's a fairly new medication in Australia, but has been used in North America for some time. New drugs can sometimes work well initially, but their effect then seems to wear off after six months or so – what we call the 'honeymoon' effect. Zonisamide continues to work for Tilly after a year, and she's also on a dose of phenobarbitone which is doing its job at the moment.

"Her drugs have made her more sedate, and she has a big sleep in the middle of the day; sometimes by my side at the practice. Her behaviour is a little odd before a fit, and sometimes she looks at me and her brain seems less attentive – as though she's not entirely 'with it.' She used to be more agile, and she's not as quick or smart as she was, but she still loves her life and enjoys going to the park. She wears me out faster than I can wear her out!"

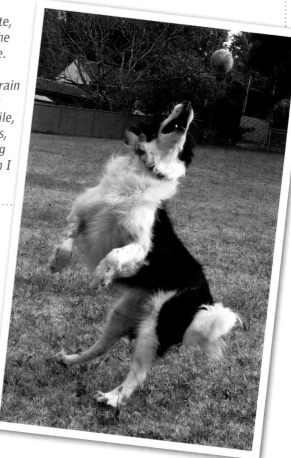

Chapter 7

Diet

The link between diet and ill-health in humans has been under the spotlight for some time now, so it's not surprising that what we feed our furry friends is also being scrutinised as never before. Some owners – and a growing number of vets – are acknowledging the connection between poor diet and a number of conditions, including epilepsy, in our animal friends.

A balance from the start

An under-nourished dog is as unhealthy as an over-fed one, so it's important to make sure we feed our dogs a balance of protein (in meat or vegetable form); fat for energy; fibre for digestion; essential fatty acids, such as omega 3 and 6, and a range of vitamins and minerals for optimum health.

The biggest favour we can do our four-legged friends is to provide them with the most nutritionally-packed diet we possibly can – from the word go.

The essentials

Dogs can produce some vitamins in their bodies, but minerals have to be obtained through diet alone, or with supplements.

Vitamins A (found in pumpkins, for example); C (in apples); D (in salmon and liver), and E (from spinach), improve the immune system and boost muscle and bone strength. The B group of vitamins, including B12 and B6, found in foods such as sweet potato, help a dog's nervous system, including her brain, to function properly.

Minerals also help to maintain the nervous system, and a lack of magnesium, manganese, selenium, calcium and zinc has been linked to seizures in some cases. Magnesium and manganese can be found in oily fish; selenium and zinc in meat, such as chicken or beef, and calcium in oily fish and yogurt.

And it's not just what your dog eats, but what he eats with it that's important, as vitamins and minerals have to work in tandem for maximum absorption and benefit.

Spices

Spices, such as turmeric and cinnamon, also play a part in maintaining good health, and could help your dog cope with the side-effects of his medication. One teaspoon of turmeric daily, sprinkled

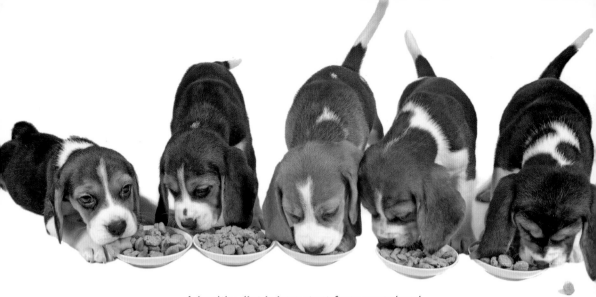

A healthy diet is important from puppyhood.

on food, is around the right amount for a Labrador, for example.

Nutritional advice

Your vet – and in some practices a nutrition nurse – should be happy to offer advice on the right diet to follow, or you could consult a canine nutritionist. If you think your dog might be deficient in any essential vitamins or minerals, you could ask your vet to run some blood tests to check this. Hair tissue mineral testing could reveal any deficiencies, too.

Supplements

As a general rule, supplements are probably not necessary if your dog's getting a balanced diet. However, if you're keen to go down the supplement route, always check with your vet beforehand, as some might react with prescribed drugs, and can be dangerous if taken in high doses. And ask your vet for their advice on which ones they'd recommend.

You might feel tempted to give your dog the same supplements you take, but dogs need to take much higher doses to gain any benefit. Supplements can be expensive

in the veterinary world, so buying yours online, rather than from your vet, could help to control costs.

Increased hunger after fitting

Most dogs love their food, and after a seizure they're usually famished, as fitting uses up a lot of energy. As long as your dog's not likely to fit again quickly (cluster), and is fully recovered, you could give her a small amount of vanilla ice cream to help raise blood sugar levels, or her regular meal.

Processed food

Pet food manufacturers have been accused of 'bulking-out' their products with less-than-healthy ingredients. If you have any concerns about feeding your dog commercial dog food which might be high in hidden additives, sugar and saturated fat, you could always check on the individual company's website to see which ingredients are used, and in what amounts.

The ketogenic diet

Devised in the US, this diet is based on high amounts of fat; sufficient protein, and very low, or no, carbohydrates, which some people – and particularly children – suffering from epilepsy have had some success with. The diet gets its name from the conversion of the high fat content of food to ketones (organic compounds that result when body fat is broken down for energy), which are then used as energy in place of carbohydrates. There's no evidence that this diet works with canine epilepsy, however, and potentially it could be harmful for dogs.

The BARF diet
The Biologically Appropriate Raw Food

(BARF) diet is based on what wolves (canis lupus), from whom dogs are descended, would have eaten in the wild: mice, for example, or larger prey if in a pack. Foods they wouldn't have come across naturally, such as dairy, soy, corn, wheat and gluten, are considered inappropriate for dogs by some.

Fans of BARF believe that, unlike commercial or cooked diets, a well-balanced raw diet, with vegetables as well as meat, allows the vitamins, minerals and enzymes in the foods to remain intact, and could reduce the amount of seizures a dog might experience as a result. Other benefits

Misty, like all dogs, loves her food.
After fitting, dogs are generally ravenous.

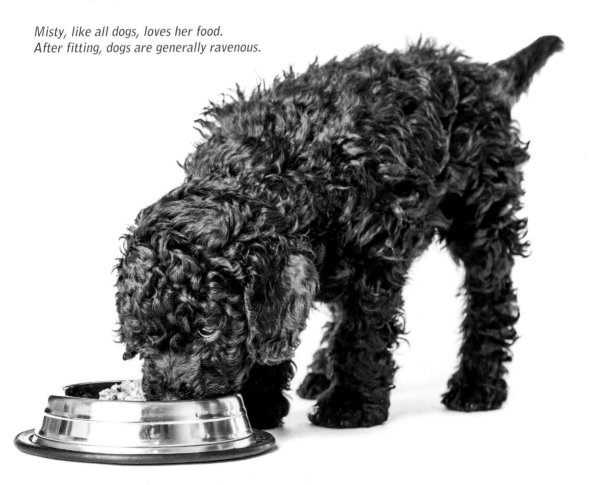

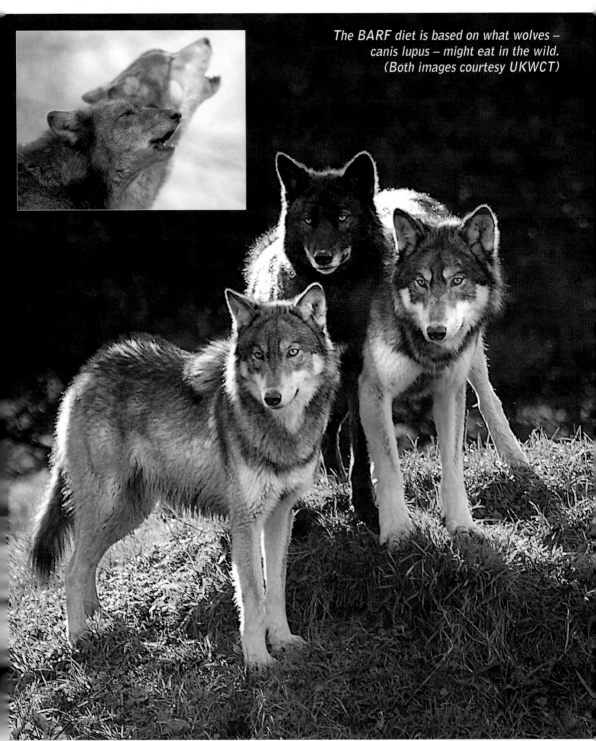

The BARF diet is based on what wolves –
canis lupus – might eat in the wild.
(Both images courtesy UKWCT)

are said to include a glossy coat; healthy skin; lean muscle tone; robust immune system; sweet-smelling breath, and more energy and vitality.

However, raw, boned meat has a greater potential for contamination, with salmonella, for example, and such a diet could be deficient in essential nutrients, as well as lead to dental health problems.

The way forward

Perhaps the answer is to lightly cook your dog's meat and vegetables to preserve as much goodness as possible, and supplement this with some high-end commercial dog food to ensure she's getting all the nutrients she needs.

If you'd rather go for 'natural' brands – like those devised by vets, say – the choice in supermarkets, pet shops, and online has never been greater.

It's also a good idea to keep your dog's diet constant without chopping and changing too much, with a few small meals throughout the day, rather than one big meal.

And, of course, your dog needs access to clean, fresh water at all times.

Healthy treats are a better option than fatty leftovers.

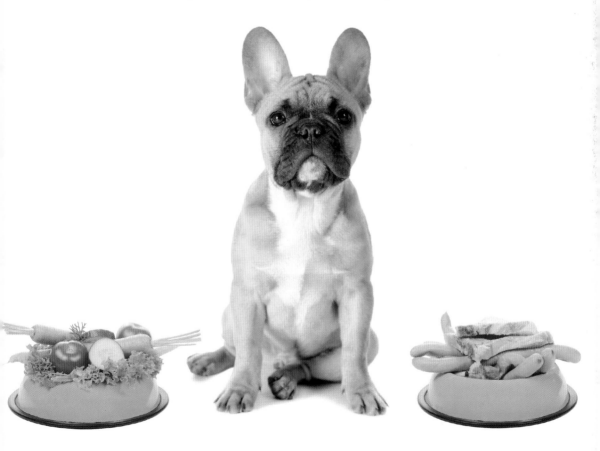

Fat and salt content

Anti-seizure medication, such as phenobarbital, stimulates appetite and increases the triglyceride (fat) level in the blood, so your dog really needs to be on a low-fat diet to help counter-balance these effects. And the sodium chloride (salt) content of your dog's diet is also relevant as it could affect the concentration of any potassium bromide she's been prescribed.

Keeping an eye on the scales

Maintaining a healthy weight is vital for every dog, and especially those coping with conditions such as epilepsy. Aim to resist your dog's doe-eyed pleas for treats and snacks, and never give her leftovers like pizza – raw carrots or strawberries are a better option. Regular exercise is also important in maintaining an appropriate weight for her size.

Case history: Sophie

Sophie, four, is owned by Lucy. She says –
"Sophie began having seizures around a year ago, and was put on phenobarbital. I wasn't happy about this, but I knew it would help to control the fits. I thought I'd do my bit too by giving her as natural a diet as possible.

"If Sophie was living a natural life in the wild, she'd be eating birds or rabbits, rather than manufactured food. I've compromised a bit, though: I give her chicken wings (from the local butcher), which I cook a little bit to kill off any bugs, just in case. She sometimes gets salmon, tuna or sardines in sunflower oil, and she loves vegetables like carrots, broccoli and sprouts. Sometimes I add turmeric or cinnamon to the chicken for flavour, which she's not so keen on, but she humours me! I also give her a small bowl of high-range pet food every day so she doesn't miss out on anything vital. She also has a late evening snack of bio-yogurt, as she loves it!

"Someone told me that grain can be a trigger for fits so I've got rid of that from her diet. I also read somewhere that peanut butter could help. We both love it!

"I think we've arrived at the best diet for her. She's not fitting as much, and seems happy enough. Her coat's great, too – nice and shiny! We'll see how it goes."

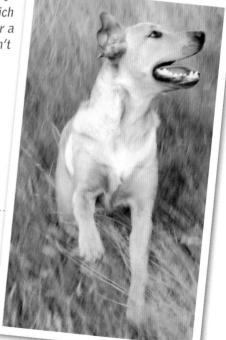

Sophie is doing well on her home-prepared diet.

Case history: Nyah

*Nyah took part in the **PDSA Pet Fit Club**, a national pet slimming competition run annually by the UK's leading veterinary charity, as she was nearly 60 per cent overweight. Her original weight gain was gradual; largely due to being fed too many treats, and having little in the way of energy because of her epilepsy medication. Nyah now weighs 50lb (23kg) after shedding just under 14lb (6.3kg).*

Her owner, Catherine, is delighted, and when Nyah's peckish now, she gives her tiny amounts of raw vegetables rather than unhealthy treats. Says Catherine: "It's been a truly amazing journey, and I can't believe the change in Nyah – she's almost unrecognisable; a completely different dog. She's a lot livelier, and is walking with a spring in her step. In the past she would lag behind me on walks, and generally had a lack of energy, but now she's up front, leading the way. She doesn't look anywhere near her 11 years now."

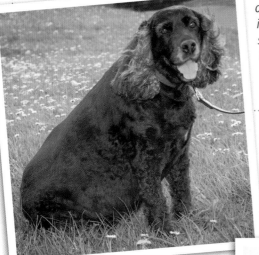

Nyah was nearly 60 per cent overweight at the start of the PDSA Pet Fit Club ...

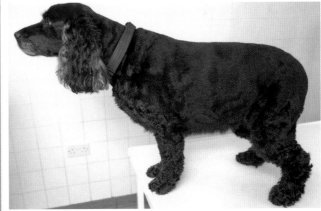

... and shed over a stone in weight.

Chapter 8

Exercise

Regular exercise is a good thing for your dog, and something you can enjoy together, so there are benefits all round. Staying active can also help your dog maintain a good weight, aid her digestion, and keep her joints and muscles supple, which is particularly important if she's suffering from other conditions, such as arthritis, as well as epilepsy.

Staying on the move

As a general rule, a few short walks a day, amounting to around an hour in total, rather than one long walk, is a good benchmark for most dogs. Every dog is different, of course, so work out what best suits yours: he'll no doubt let you know what he prefers.

If your dog seems drained of energy, perhaps as a result of the drugs he's taking for his seizures, it makes sense to reduce walking time until he feels perkier. And if his fits are due to low blood sugar, or heart disease, have a word with your vet about the level of exercise that would be appropriate for him.

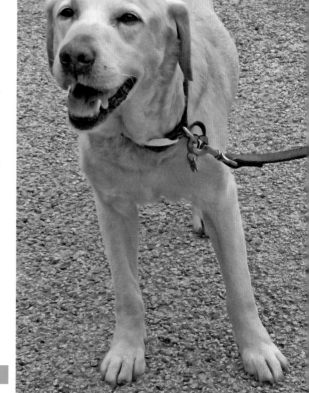

Monty loves going for walks ...

could also help cool him down after a fit. Of course, some dogs are exhausted after a seizure, and just want to sleep, so be guided by your dog to a large extent.

The importance of play
Exercise through play – on the beach, in the park or at home – is a good bonding experience, as well as fun for you both. Play will also help to keep your dog mentally stimulated and ready to enjoy life, despite her epilepsy.

Ataxia
Anti-seizure medications, particularly given in high doses, can lead to ataxia – co-ordination and hind leg problems – causing your dog to wobble or stagger around. While it's important for your dog to take enough exercise to keep his muscles and joints strong and flexible, if

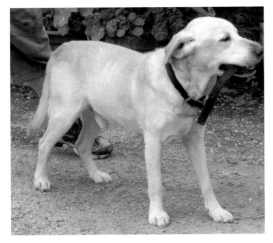

... and leading the way.

Calming effect
If your dog paces after a seizure, or is particularly nervous, a leisurely walk might help to calm him, and being outside

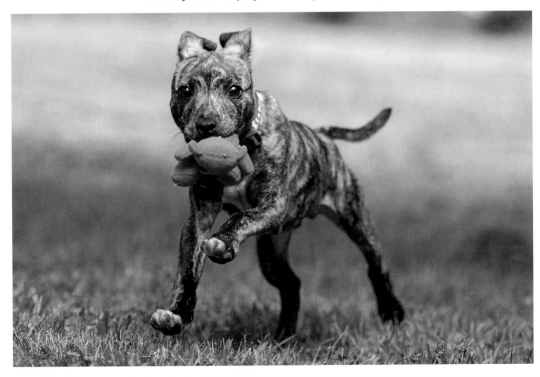

Murray loves to play. (Courtesy Clint Images)

he's affected by ataxia it's probably best to go at a slower, steadier pace until he's confident on all four paws again.

You could ask your vet to refer you to a veterinary physiotherapist to see if they can recommend exercises to help to strengthen the muscles in your dog's legs; improve co-ordination, and help avoid any ligament damage.

Exercise in the water

Many dog breeds, but especially Spaniels, Terriers and Labradors, love being in the water, and having epilepsy shouldn't preclude your dog from getting his paws wet.

As a general rule, by working with your vet (who will have to refer your dog for hydrotherapy) and the therapist, hydrotherapy should be a good, all-round experience for your dog.

IMPORTANT CONSIDERATIONS

Most hydrotherapists are happy to treat dogs with epilepsy as long as the condition is under control, and a dog hasn't had one or more seizures in the week prior to the hydrotherapy session. If your dog's over-anxious or nervous, or if being in water is a stressful, rather than an enjoyable, experience for him, hydro might not be the right route to take. And whether there's a risk that light reflecting on the water in the pool could trigger a reaction in your dog, should also be taken into account.

ALL-ROUND FITNESS

Hydro can help to strengthen and tone muscles, increase muscle bulk, and relieve joint pain, swelling and stiffness. Warm water also increases the circulation of blood to the muscles, helping them relax, and boosts the supply of oxygen and nutrients to the tissues. It also helps to flush away waste products, and improves

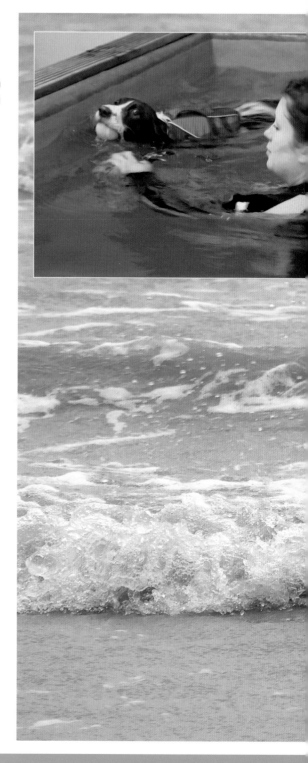

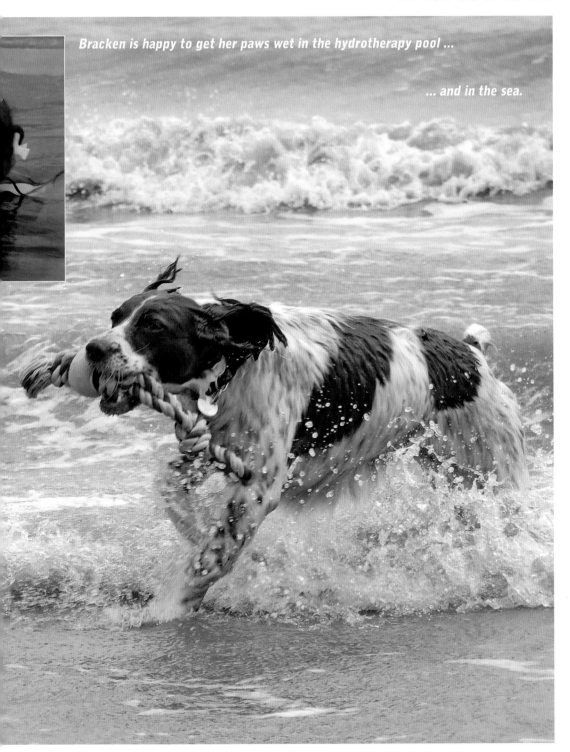

Bracken is happy to get her paws wet in the hydrotherapy pool ...

... and in the sea.

hind-leg co-ordination, so there are a number of physiological benefits to hydrotherapy for dogs whose epilepsy is under control.

Mood enhancer

Hydrotherapy can have a positive effect on your dog's mood, and help to reduce the stress she could well be experiencing as a result of her epilepsy. Hydro can provide mental stimulation, too, and some dogs can be quite perky when they leave the pool. Generally speaking, there's usually an overall improvement in a dog's mental state within a couple of weeks of starting hydrotherapy.

First steps

During the initial consultation your therapist will want to know which type of epilepsy your dog is suffering from; the average length of her seizures, and her behaviour before and after a fit. You might also be asked for an up-to-date list of the medication your dog is taking, and the result of the last blood test (or the therapist might ask your vet for this information).

Your dog will be given a head-to-tail examination, and her muscle mass measurements will be taken. She will be showered before she goes on the water-walker, or into the pool, and then dried by hand, or blow dried – which some dogs like, although most tolerate, rather than enjoy this. Ideally, your dog should be assessed before and after each swim, with temperature checks taken, as dogs can suffer heat exhaustion more quickly than humans.

A typical session

Most hydrotherapy centres provide a pool, rather like a large fish tank, and an aquatic treadmill, or water-walker. A treadmill is

Your dog could have his hydro sessions on a water-walker or in the pool. (Courtesy CHA)

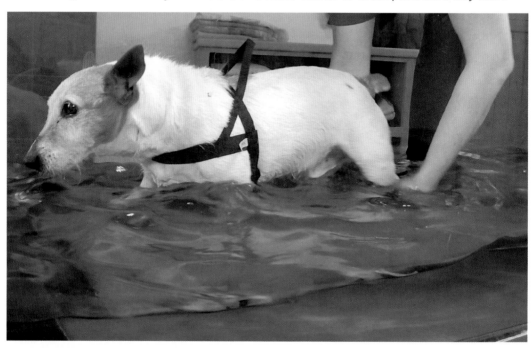

Case study: Mylo

Mylo, who's 7, is owned by Louise, a hydrotherapist at Chief Glen in Kent. Louise says –
"Mylo was just over two years old when he had his first epileptic seizure. He was
diagnosed with idiopathic epilepsy, and put on phenobarbitone (pb). At the beginning,
Mylo was very ataxic and lethargic, sleeping more or less all the time. He was switched to
a lower dose of pb, and then potassium bromide was added. He still has seizures every so
often, but they're less violent now and don't last as long. He was also diagnosed with hip
and elbow dysplasia when he was 7 months old, so he was already coping with a joint issue,
then with ataxia from the epilepsy drugs which made him less mobile.

"Mylo still lives life to the full, though. He likes to play and go for walks, and he loves
being in the water. He has hydrotherapy sessions once a week, and I believe the treatment
helps to strengthen his muscles; keep him mobile, and increase his stamina. With the
improvements to his circulation that hydro brings, I find Mylo's very relaxed after his
session, which I believe helps to reduce stress levels, and in turn helps his epilepsy. I think
he gains both mentally and physically, and it's nice to see Mylo enjoying hydrotherapy,
knowing the full benefits which it brings to him."

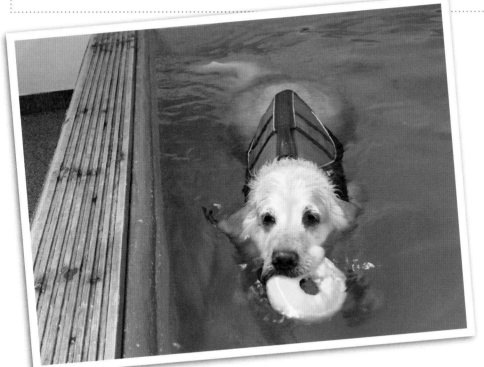

Mylo is benefiting from his sessions in the pool.

considered safer than a pool for dogs with epilepsy, as they can be better monitored, and the water could be drained quickly, and the dog supported, should there be a fitting incident. It's usually a better option for small dogs, too.

However, many epileptic dogs, particularly medium and larger sized breeds, can go in the pool, with a therapist alongside for encouragement, and as a precautionary measure. Dogs will usually wear a life jacket or a harness on the treadmill, and in the pool.

Time in the water

Sessions usually start gradually, and can increase quite quickly for some dogs, although those who are overweight will probably take it slower. Although your dog shouldn't be pushed, if she's coping well with the treatment, it's advisable to take her for therapy twice a week for the first two weeks, as once a week would take longer to show any benefit. Your therapist will be able to guide you on this.

Once a week in the long term should be all your dog needs. Some insurance companies will pay for a maximum ten sessions only, so do check your policy first, or be prepared to fund more sessions yourself. (As a rough guide, a full session of around 30 minutes, will cost in the region of £30).

Feedback

After the first session the therapist will request feedback from you about how your dog has responded to the treatment: for example, was she stiff or tired afterwards (which might indicate she's overdone it in her first session), and has her mood improved?

As her owner you should go by your instincts. If you think something's wrong, or you don't think your dog would benefit from further sessions, discuss this with the therapist and adjustments can be made. After the tenth session your vet will be given a full report on what improvements in your dog's overall condition there have been.

Trained therapists

Hydrotherapy is not as well regulated as it should be, so it's advisable, particularly with an epileptic dog, to use a centre that is registered with the Canine Hydrotherapy Association (CHA), or with NARCH (National Association of Registered Canine Hydrotherapists). Most pet insurance companies will only pay out for hydro practised by a therapist registered with one of these organisations.

Chapter 9

Complementary therapies

Complementary therapies could help to reduce the side-effects of conventional treatments, and improve your dog's quality of life. Some owners believe certain therapies actually extend their dogs' lives. They're designed to work alongside conventional treatments – not replace them – and while most therapies can certainly help in the majority of cases, they can't alter the course of your dog's epilepsy – or provide a cure, sadly.

While they're generally safe if practised by a qualified therapist from a recognised organisation, a veterinary referral is usually needed. Some therapies are given singly; others in combination with another treatment. The following are some of the popular ones –

Acupuncture

Acupuncture is based on the Chinese art of gently moving energy (chi) around the body. Fine needles are inserted through the skin at certain points to help relieve pain (the therapy stimulates the release of the body's own pain-relieving and anti-inflammatory substances), and to promote general well-being.

It can be slightly uncomfortable for your dog when the needles are inserted, but shouldn't hurt – some even doze off during a session, which usually lasts around 30 minutes. Some therapists use low-level lasers instead of needles.

Acupuncture can only be performed by a vet, although acupressure (using fingertips and no needles) can be practised on a dog by anyone qualified to do so. Studies into the benefits of acupuncture have shown it can be effective in helping to reduce the number of seizures in some cases.

Bach flower therapy

This therapy is named after Dr Edward Bach, who drew on the healing properties of flowers to create 38 different essences corresponding to a patient's particular emotional state.

Some owners have found that Bach Rescue Remedy is effective when their dog is about to have a seizure, or as an overall stress reducer to help prevent further seizures. The essence can be dropped directly into your dog's mouth, or diluted in his drinking water.

Canine Bowen Technique

This is a light touch, soft tissue therapy named after its innovator, Tom Bowen, which was adapted around ten years ago for use on dogs. The therapist gently moves his fingers over muscle, ligaments and tendons on various parts of a dog's body to promote healing and pain relief.

Galen Canine Myotherapy

This dedicated hands-on treatment targets muscle pain and mobility issues originating from trauma or repetitive strain. The therapy has had some success in extending the period between seizures.

Homoeopathy

Homoeopathy is based on the principle of 'like is cured by like.' Where conventional

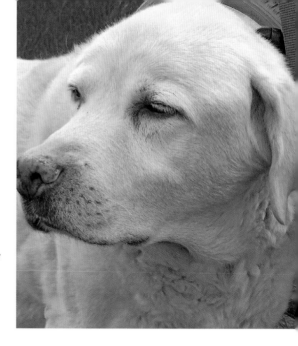

Dexter, 15, who's owned by Clare, has been epileptic since he was 17 months old. After being referred to a homoeopathic vet for therapy, however, he has been free of grand mal seizures for at least six years.

medicine suppresses symptoms, homeopathy provokes the body into healing itself. Commonly prescribed remedies include belladonna, aconitum, and, in cases of vaccine-related seizures, thuja.

Reiki

Reiki (pronounced 'ray key') is Japanese for Universal Life Energy. It's a natural, safe, and simple hands-on healing method with no manipulation involved. It's believed that reiki creates and promotes self-healing, balances energies, and revitalises. Dogs generally become calm and relaxed during treatment.

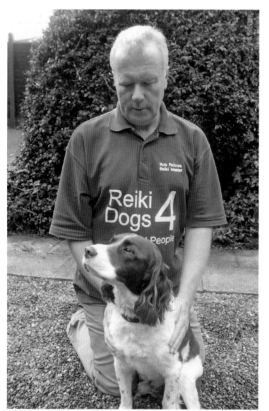

Monty receiving treatment from Rob Fellows, International Reiki Master.

Case history: Taggart

Taggart was owned by Canine Bowen therapists Sally and Ron. Says Sally –

"Taggart had his first seizure when he was three. He went on to suffer isolated fits followed by clusters, and was put on phenobarbital. He was also diagnosed as hypothyroid (under-active thyroid). With our background in animal behaviour, and as canine Bowen specialists, we decided to do what we could to help control the seizures, or at least give Taggart a better quality of life.

"There seemed to be a pattern of muscle tension immediately prior to seizure, and after seizure the muscles are even tighter. With the agreement of our vet, we used Canine Bowen Technique at intervals of every 6-8weeks (or sooner if we noticed early signs of problems with Taggart), and found we were able to relax the muscles and thus, apparently, were able to avert the build-up to Taggart's seizures. Simultaneously, we changed Taggart's diet to a mixture of commercial and home-prepared food, with added nutritional therapy to counteract any mineral imbalance.

"The results of this plan were stunning, and within four to five months the seizures had stopped. After two months of no seizures, and with our vet's agreement, we began to slowly wean Taggart off his phenobarbital. He had one minor cluster of seizures, and then no more. Taggart lived until he was eleven years old without any further need for epilepsy medication."

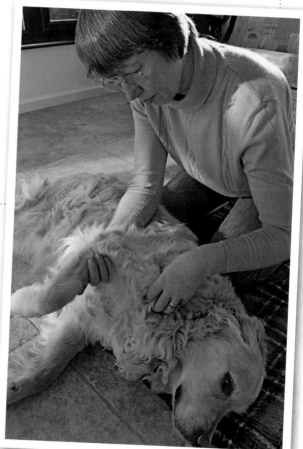

Taggart receiving treatment from Sally.
(Courtesy Ron Askew EGCBT)

Case history: Harry and Merlin

Uncle and nephew, Harry and Merlin, are owned by Sally. She says –

"Harry had his first seizure when he was two (he's now 8), and as time went on his seizures began occurring closer together: around every six weeks or so. I've always been anti-medication, and prefer a natural approach to medicine, so I changed his diet to a grain-free one, also free of certain meats, and he went 3 months before his next seizure. He's now on a raw diet and goes 4-6 months without a fit. I also give him skullcap and valerian on a daily basis, which definitely helps with the frequency.

"Merlin was having severe, frequent seizures and I felt helpless, as he was already having the same diet as Harry, and was also taking the supplement Epitaur – a combination of taurine, tyrosine, magnesium, zinc, and vitamin B, which I believe many epileptic dogs are deficient in. I started him on some herbal supplements, but he continued to have seizures every 2-4 weeks.

"He then had a consultation with a homeopathic vet on his 4th birthday, and was given some remedies. The following afternoon he began having recurrent seizures. This all happened on the Tuesday; his remedies didn't arrive until the Thursday, and by Friday I was so worried I took him to the vet for a blood test (which was normal), and discussed putting him on medication as we couldn't continue as we were. This was a massive decision for me: I felt defeated, and was not happy about him needing the meds.

"We had a good night that night, so I decided to hold off with the meds to see if the homeopathy worked. We were given two different remedies: one for 3 days, followed by one for 7 days – and then asked to report back to the homeopathic vet a week later. She was pleased with our progress, and so, assuming there are no more seizures, we have decided to do a split dose in another 3 weeks' time (one tablet in the evening, followed by one the following morning, just for those two days), then wait a month and report back again.

"It's early days, but I'm pleased we've stayed off the meds so far. I'll always do what I feel is best for Merlin, and would never let him suffer, but medication will be a last resort."

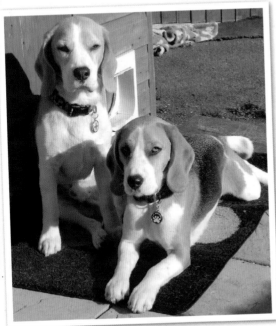

The Beagle boys: Harry and Merlin.

Case history: Samson

Samson, owned by Sue, is being treated by vet Richard Allport of the Natural Medicine Centre in Hertfordshire. Says Richard –

"I first met Samson in June 2010 when he was five years old, and had been fitting for two years. The fits were becoming more frequent and more intense.

"Samson was in good general health and his blood tests were normal. After his second fit, phenobarbitone had been dispensed, but it had been decided to discontinue this because of the risk of adverse effects, and to give no anticonvulsant treatment unless the situation deteriorated.

"It did, and Samson was brought along to me to see if natural medicines could provide reasonable control of the epilepsy. I have been using natural medicines – including herbs, homoeopathy, acupuncture, and nutritional supplements – for thirty years, and in that time have seen very good results with treating epileptic patients.

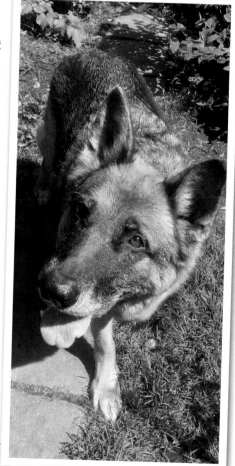

"During the consultation I discussed every aspect of Samson: his character; his likes and dislikes; medical history; sleep patterns; when and where the seizures happened; how long they lasted; how long he took to recover, and what position his head and limbs were in during fits. All these questions and many more were necessary to make sure I could formulate an individual prescription of herbs, homoeopathic medicines and supplements that would have a chance of controlling the condition.

"I dispensed a course of herbal Skullcap and Valerian combination; an amino acid and vitamin supplement, and four homoeopathic medicines, all for long term treatment. Samson subsequently had four fits, but these seemed less severe than before, and he had no more until December, which augured well. It is not unusual for natural therapies to take a while to begin to work at their best, so I hadn't been worried by the fact that Samson had had a few fits after beginning treatment. More improvement followed, and from 2011 to date (February 2014), Samson has had only three fits. He's living proof that natural medicines are able to prevent seizures – and with none of the adverse effects of conventional medication."

Samson is benefiting from his treatment.

Case history: Moon

Moon, five, was treated by Galen Canine Myotherapist Julia Robertson, of the Galen Therapy Centre in West Sussex. Says Susan, Moon's owner –

"Moon was diagnosed with severe vaccine damage at ten weeks old, leaving him with epilepsy, among other problems. He was treated homeopathically to reverse some of the effects of the vaccine, and then began myotherapy: initially to ease some of the physical stresses on his body.

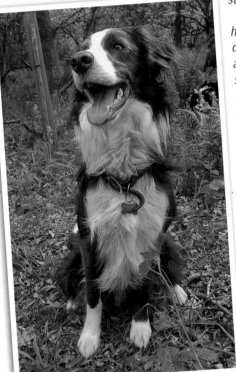

"The difference in Moon is quite dramatic: he has gone from being totally emotionally 'shut down,' with a high frequency of focal seizures and an inability to interact with people, strange situations and other dogs, to being on a low maintenance dose of medication, and almost seizure-free. With regular myotherapy he can now be touched; is happy to greet strangers and friends; is playful, energetic, and full of mischief, and able to think and react to instructions."

Moon is clearly on the mend.

Chapter 10

When euthanasia is the only option

When your dog's quality of life is so reduced, with the bad days far outweighing the good ones, the time has probably come to release her from the pain and unhappiness she's possibly feeling. Of course, this is not a decision to rush into, which is likely to be one of the hardest – and saddest – you'll ever have to make.

When the time's right

There are usually tell-tale signs that will let you know when your dog's finding his symptoms of epilepsy more than he can bear. He'll probably be eating and drinking less, and might not want to play, or go for walks with you, as before: in essence, he'll be withdrawing. With help and advice from your vet, you can do the kindest thing for your dog, and let him go.

Letting go

Dogs have a special way of letting us know when they've had enough; often just by the way they look at us. Sometimes they hang on because they're worried we won't be able to cope on our own when they've gone.

So to help your dog, you could say something to her along the lines of: 'I'll miss you so much when you've gone, but I can't watch you in so much pain anymore. I think you'd like to be set free.' With this 'permission' from those she loves the most, she'll feel able to take her leave of the family.

Euthanasia procedure

Euthanasia is considered a peaceful and quick death; almost a 'good' death, if such a thing is possible. Generally speaking, the process involves an intravenous injection of barbiturates into a limb, with death typically occurring within 30 seconds.

Your vet might give your dog an initial injection to make her unconscious, to give you a chance to say a final goodbye, before a second injection will put her to sleep. (If you want to be present, chat with your vet beforehand so you know what to expect). Some vets are happy to carry out the procedure at your home instead, which might be less upsetting for you and your dog.

A final resting place

If you can, decide early on if you'd prefer

a cremation or a burial for your dog, either at home or in a pet cemetery. It's a very personal decision, and really only yours to make. Your vet should be able to recommend a company in your area, or you could contact the Association of Private Pet Cemeteries and Crematoria (APPCC).

If you choose to bury your dog's remains in your own garden – perhaps wrapped in his favourite blanket, rather than anything plastic to assist the natural decaying process – it's best to check first with your local authority, in case there are any objections.

Although a burial at a pet cemetery wouldn't be as personal (and is usually a more expensive option), everything is done for you if you can't face doing it yourself. And by choosing this route, you can always visit your dog's grave, even if you move house.

Another option is to keep your dog's ashes at home with you: perhaps in a wooden or cast resin casket.

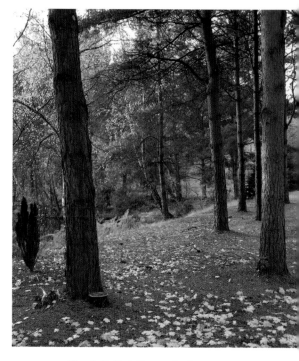

Norfolk Pet Crematorium.

Coping with your loss

There's no right or wrong way to grieve. Give yourself time to mourn, and don't admonish yourself for being upset about your dog's death – only you know what she meant to you and your family.

It'll help to remember the good times you had with your dog, but if you're finding you need extra support dealing with your loss, you could contact the Pet Bereavement Support Service (PBSS), run by the Blue Cross animal charity. It provides emotional support and practical information for pet owners through its confidential telephone service.

There are various ways you could thank your dog for the good times you shared: perhaps by posting an 'in memory' notice on a dedicated website, such as Living With Pet Bereavement or Rainbow Bridge;

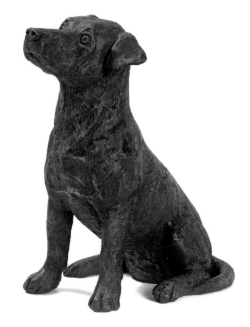

(Courtesy Petributes)

other sites might make a small charge for a similar service. You could also consider making a donation to a pet charity, or a local rescue centre, in your dog's memory.

Case history: Wally

Wally was owned by Rick, who established the non-profit Wally Canine Epilepsy Foundation in Delaware, USA, in honour of his dog. Says Rick –

"Wally was diagnosed with idiopathic epilepsy a few months shy of his third birthday. He was put on phenobarbital and potassium bromide liquid, but continued having seizures, including multiple clusters. The end result was significant neurological damage that was progressive.

"On January 29, 2013, our family decided that Wally's quality of life was deteriorating rapidly, as was his physical and mental health, and arranged to have him euthanized. Wally was shown all the love and compassion any dog could ever ask for – he was allowed to eat all the pizza, ice cream, ham, and tuna casserole he could possibly want – and a few days later we helped Wally cross the Rainbow Bridge to be free of this terrible disease.

"After Wally's passing, there was a terrible void in our home. Not only was a 170lb dog the size of a sofa no longer present, but the sudden decrease in stress levels, and not having to adhere to a strict medication ritual twice a day, only seemed to magnify the loss. As a family we decided we wanted a fitting tribute and memorial to Wally. He was a big dog with a big heart and a big personality, who loved others unconditionally."

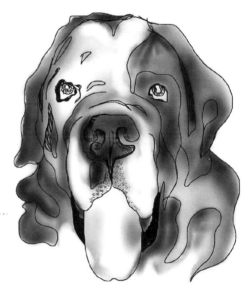

Wally, who inspired a foundation.

Case history: Daisy

Daisy was owned by Barbara, who says –

"Daisy had her first fit shortly after her third birthday, followed by cluster seizures. She then had a serious episode when she began fitting at 11pm and couldn't stop. We took her to the vet at midnight and the fitting was eventually controlled at 1.30am. This could have been fatal.

"From that time her medication was regularly increased, and she was on phenobarbital, potassium bromide and Keppra®. This drug regime was successful for three months until she started fitting again, more and more frequently. She then became generally unwell: not eating, and not wanting to go for walks.

"The vet had been very supportive throughout the progress of her condition, and, as soon as the severity of it became apparent, discussed with us the probable outcome. We all agreed that the most important factor was Daisy's quality of life. Once her liver had become damaged by the medication we were advised to gradually wean her off the tablets, and just treat the fits as they occurred, with the understanding that this would only work for a short period.

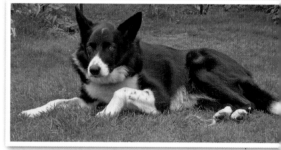

Daisy.

"When the final fit started and it wasn't possible to stop it, we phoned the vets and asked to have Daisy put to sleep. They were very kind and opened the surgery early on a Saturday morning to help us. I was grateful that our vets were honest with us about Daisy's condition so that we were semi-prepared for what happened and didn't have false hope.

"Although we always knew there would be no happy outcome for Daisy, it was still very distressing to lose her. I felt particularly bad that she had only managed to have four years of life. Before the epilepsy she was such a healthy, lively dog, and it seemed so sad that she had so few years. Our two previous dogs had been buried in our garden, but as Daisy was quite a lot bigger, and I have a horror of foxes digging up a body in a too-shallow grave, she was cremated.

"We scattered her ashes on a local beach, in the nearby woods, and in our garden – her favourite places. We planted a deutzia in the garden in her memory, and for my next birthday my husband commissioned a portrait of Daisy, which hangs in our sitting room. It took several months for us to come to terms with Daisy's death, and then we started to look around for a new friend, and eventually found Hal, a rescue dog, who's a delight and has helped us a lot."

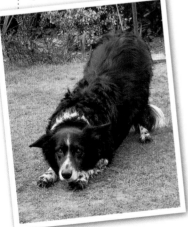

Hal the rescue dog, helping to heal.

Case history: Brody

Brody was owned by Kristen, a volunteer for North East Rottweiler Rescue, which has centres across New England, USA. Says Kristen –

"Brody lived a pretty healthy life until just before his fourth birthday when he had his first seizure, followed by another one a month later. We tried various medications, including potassium bromide, replaced later by Keppra®, zonisamide, and phenobarbitone, but the seizures continued. Sometimes, he could have psycho motor seizures where he would climb walls or just race to a wall and try to climb it: so scary! We were already resigned to gating him in a bedroom by himself during the day, but he still ended up cutting himself on a lamp he broke during a seizure.

"In the end we were trying everything: Chinese herbs, changing his food, changing his meds, and reiki, which we did together. He was a difficult case for sure, but he was always a perfect gentleman.

"Then things started to fall apart. He developed extreme ataxia to the point he couldn't walk, and a large mass, which was probably cancer, showed up on an x-ray.

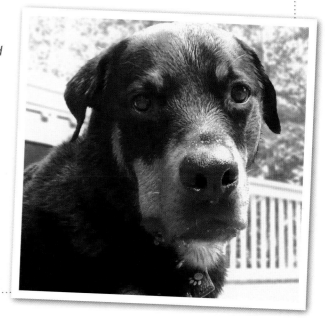

"The vet suggested we spoil him and let him go when the time came, so we made the horrible decision to put him down the next day after giving him the best 24 hours we could: he had donuts, steak, and ice cream. He walked into the vet on his own, and he passed with his favourite toy, his ball, in his mouth. He was only 7 years, 7 months old.

"I feel we did the best we could for him. We pulled out all the stops, but in the end we couldn't save him. I wear a cremation bead, with Brody's ashes in it, every day. He's always close to my heart, and always will be."

Chapter 11

Conclusion

Receiving the news that your dog has epilepsy is upsetting, and not something you ever wanted to hear, or had expected to have to cope with. Epilepsy can be debilitating for your dog, and will take some time to adjust to – for you and him.

On a positive note, there's a lot that can be done to relieve your faithful friend's suffering, including drug treatments, lifestyle adjustments, and complementary therapies. And putting your dog on a low-fat diet, however hard that might be for you both to stomach, can help to manage his epilepsy, and, ultimately, keep him as healthy as possible to better deal with the condition.

Hopefully, the case histories featured in this book have demonstrated that a diagnosis of epilepsy doesn't have to be the end of your dog's world – or yours. The fun things you've always loved to do together don't have to be tossed aside like old bones. By making some adjustments around the home to reduce the likelihood of injury during a seizure, and by reducing the stress your dog experiences where possible, you're taking steps to manage the condition as effectively as possible.

It's important to work with your vet for the best possible outcome for your hound. If your dog's not responding well to treatment, or if you're worried about the side-effects of some of the available drugs, don't be afraid to ask your vet for help, advice, and an opportunity to discuss alternative, less toxic, therapies. Your dog will thank you for it from the tips of his paws to the end of her tail.

And while conventional treatment options might seem limited at the moment – and largely centred on trying, not always successfully, to reduce seizure frequency, rather than providing a cure – take heart that research is under way into the role genes play in epilepsy. There's always the hope that gene-based therapy, alongside responsible breeding, could eradicate the condition one day.

In the meantime, don't despair about your dog's epilepsy: there's every reason to believe she'll carry on living her life more or less as before. After all, she doesn't know she's epileptic, and just wants to enjoy being a dog. However hard it might be, try and let her do just that!

Chapter 12

Useful contacts and further reading

Veterinary

Small Animal Specialist Hospital (SASH)
Sydney, Australia
www.sashvets.com

The Animal Health Trust
www.aht.org.uk
http://www.aht.org.uk/cms-display/
genetics_cares.html

Royal Veterinary College (RVC)
www.rvc.ac.uk

British Veterinary Association
www.bva.co.uk

British Small Animal Veterinary Association
(BSAVA)
www.bsava.com

Southpaws Speciality Surgery for Animals
www.southpaws.com.au

Willows Veterinary Centre & Referral
Services
www.willows.net.uk

Complementary

Holisticvet Ltd
www.holisticvet.co.uk

Canine Bowen Technique
www.caninebowentechnique.com
rainbowdogsschool@btinternet.com

The Natural Medicine Centre
www.naturalmedicinecentre.co.uk

The Galen Therapy Centre & Foundation for
Canine Studies
www.galentherapycentre.co.uk
www.caninetherapy.co.uk

Association of British Veterinary
Acupuncturists (ABVA)
www.abva.co.uk

British Association of Homoeopathic
Veterinary Surgeons (BAHVS)
www.bahvs.com

Canine Hydrotherapy Association (CHA)
www.canine-hydrotherapy.org

National Association of Registered Canine Hydrotherapists (NARCH)
www.narch.org.uk

Chiefglen K9 Training School
www.chiefglenK9hydrotherapy.co.uk

Reiki4dogs
www.RobFellowsReiki.com/reiki-for-dogs

Hawksmoor Hydrotherapy
www.hawksmoorhydrotherapy.com

Trusts, clubs and charities

The Kennel Club
(The UK's largest organisation dedicated to the health & welfare of dogs)
www.thekennelclub.org.uk

Petsavers
(The charitable division of the British Small Animal Veterinary Association)
www.petsavers.org.uk

PDSA
(A veterinary charity caring for pet patients belonging to people in need)
www.pdsa.org.uk
www.pdsa.org.uk/petfitclub

Pets as Therapy
(Volunteers with registered PAT dogs visit people in hospitals & homes)
www.petsastherapy.org

Battersea Dogs & Cats Home
www.battersea.org.uk

The Karlton Index
(Measuring the health of pedigree dogs)
www.thekarltonindex.com

The Phyllis Croft Foundation for canine epilepsy
www.pcfce.org.uk

Dogs Trust
(The UK's largest dog welfare charity)
www.dogstrust.org.uk

Medical Detection Dogs
www.medicaldetectiondogs.org.uk

Dogs Lost
(Reuniting lost dogs with their owners)
www.doglost.co.uk

Pet Log
(The UK's largest lost and found database for microchipped pets)
www.petlog.org.uk

The Retired Greyhound Trust
www.retiredgreyhounds.co.uk

Animal Aiders
(Canine first-aid courses)
www.animalaiders.co.uk

Dogtor John
(Food intolerances in dogs and people)
www.dogtorJ.com

North East Rottweiler Rescue & Referral
www.rottrescue.org

Cocker Spaniel Rescue of BC
www.csrbc.org

Online sites for prescription treatments, supplements, vet and pet products and other services

www.vet-medic.com
www.animeddirect.co.uk
www.VetUK.co.uk
www.furrypharm.co.uk
www.petdrugsonline.co.uk
www.vmd.defra.gov.uk
www.vmd.gov.uk
www.medaust.com
www.petspec.co.uk

www.petelements.co.uk
www.healthforanimals.co.uk
www.tuffies.co.uk
www.ancol.co.uk
www.animal-magix.co.uk
www.allaboutdogfood.co.uk
www.petlifeonline.co.uk
www.boneandrag.com
www.yappersandbarkersonline.co.uk
www.petmeds.co.uk
www.viovet.co.uk
www.forum.hmedicine.com
www.chihuahuahotel.com

Crematoria/loss/remembrance

Norfolk Pet Crematorium Ltd
www.norfolkpetcrematorium.com

Dignity Pet Crematorium
www.dignitypetcrem.co.uk

Association of Private Pet Cemeteries
& Crematoria (APPCC)
www.appcc.org.uk

Blue Cross
(Pet bereavement support service)
Tel: 0800 096 6606
www.bluecross.org.uk

Living with Pet Bereavement
www.livingwithpetbereavement.com

Rainbow Bridge
www.rainbowbridge.com

Petributes
www.petributes.co.uk

Vets2Home
In-home pet end-of-life and euthanasia
www.vets2home.co.uk

The UK Wolf Conservation Trust
www.ukwct.org.uk

Magazines

Dogs Today
Tel: 01276 858880
www.dogstodaymagazine.co.uk

Dogs Monthly
www.dogsmonthly.co.uk

Your Dog
www.yourdog.co.uk

Dogs Life
www.dogslife.com.au

Forums & social networking sites

www.mypetonline.co.uk
www.K9friendsunited.com
www.petforums.co.uk

Events

Crufts
(Kennel Club event at NEC Birmingham)
www.crufts.org.uk

Discover Dogs Show
(Kennel Club event in London)
www.discoverdogs.org.uk

The London Pet Show
www.londonpetshow.co.uk

All About Dogs
Aztec Events
(Shows in Newbury, Newark, Lincoln,
Suffolk & Norfolk)
www.allaboutdogsshow.co.uk

The foregoing information was correct
at the time of going to press, and no
responsibility is taken for omission or error.
Inclusion does not confer endorsement by
the author or publisher.

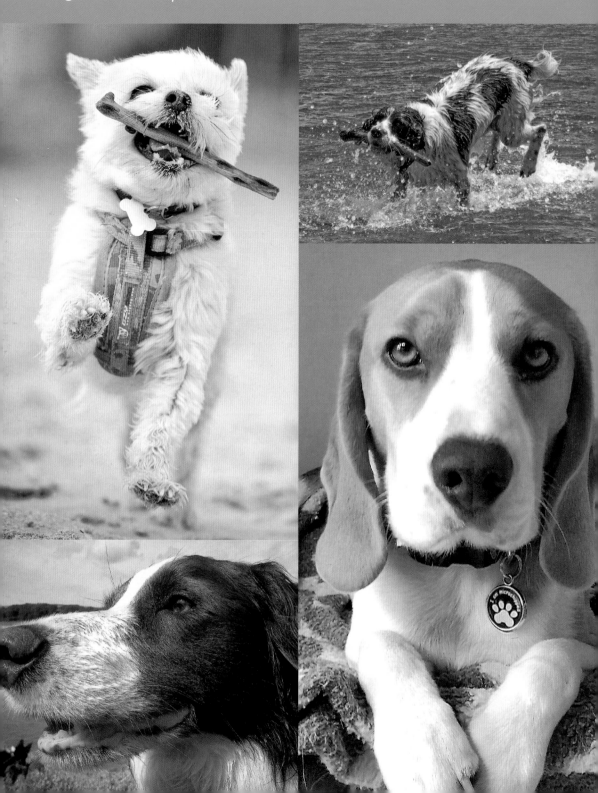

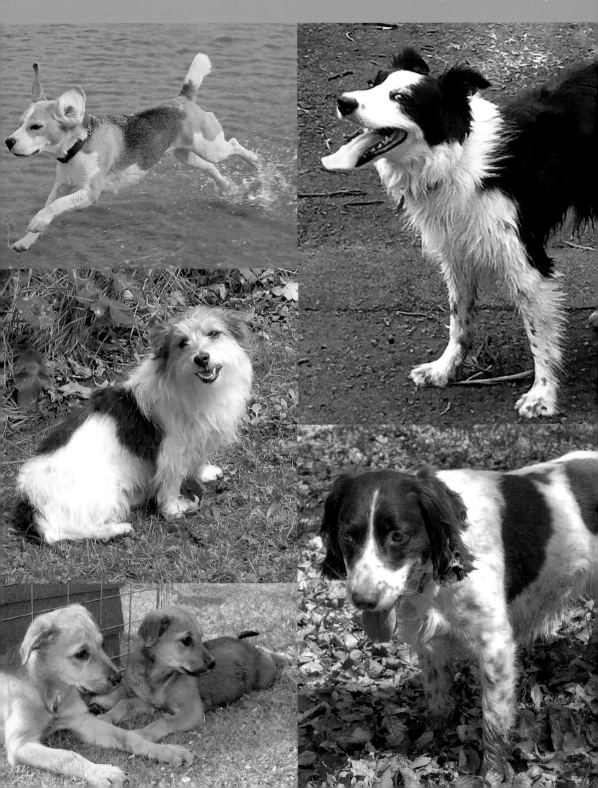

Index

Visit Hubble and Hattie on the web: www.hubbleandhattie.com & www.hubbleandhattie.blogspot.co.uk
• Details of all books • Special offers • Newsletter • New book news

79

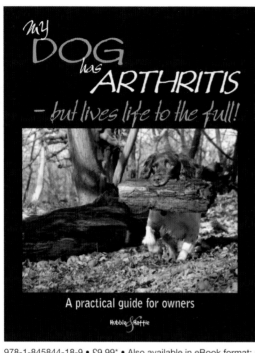

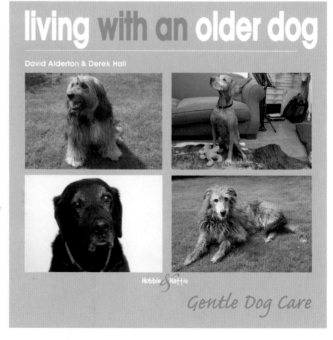